Nebraska Symposium on Motivation

Volume 57

Series Editor
Debra A. Hope
Lincoln, Nebraska, USA

For further volumes, go to
http://www.springer.com/series/7596

Gustavo Carlo · Lisa J. Crockett ·
Miguel A. Carranza

Editors

Health Disparities in Youth and Families

Research and Applications

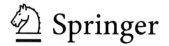 Springer

Editors
Gustavo Carlo
Department of Psychology
University of Nebraska
Lincoln, NE 68588-0308, USA
gcarlo1@unl.edu

Lisa J. Crockett
Department of Psychology
University of Nebraska
Lincoln, NE 68588-0308, USA
ecrockett1@unl.edu

Miguel A. Carranza
Department of Sociology
University of Nebraska
Lincoln, NE 68588-0324, USA
mcarranza1@unl.edu

ISSN 0146-7875
ISBN 978-1-4419-7091-6   e-ISBN 978-1-4419-7092-3
DOI 10.1007/978-1-4419-7092-3
Springer New York Dordrecht Heidelberg London

Library of Congress Control Number: 2010936341

Printed on acid-free paper

Springer is part of Springer Science+Business Media (www.springer.com)

Preface

The volume editors for this 57th volume of the Nebraska Symposium on Motivation are Gustavo Carlo, Lisa Crockett and Miguel Carranza. The volume editors coordinated the symposium that lead to this volume including selecting and inviting the contributors. My thanks go to the Gus, Lisa and Miguel and to our contributors for outstanding presentations and chapters. This interdisciplinary work on health disparities is a proud addition to this historic series.

This Symposium series is supported by funds provided by the Chancellor of the University of Nebraska-Lincoln, Harvey Perlman, and by funds given in memory of Professor Harry K. Wolfe to the University of Nebraska Foundation by the late Professor Cora L. Friedline. We are extremely grateful for the Chancellor's generous support of the Symposium series and for the University of Nebraska Foundation's support via the Friedline bequest. This symposium volume, like those in the recent past, is dedicated to the memory of Professor Wolfe, who brought psychology to the University of Nebraska. After studying with Professor Wilhelm Wundt, Professor Wolfe returned to this, his native state, to establish the first undergraduate laboratory in psychology in the nation. As a student at Nebraska, Professor Friedline studied psychology under Professor Wolfe.

Debra A. Hope
University of Nebraska-Lincoln, USA
Series Editor

Contents

Contributors

Gustavo Carlo Department of Psychology, University of Nebraska, Lincoln, NE, USA, gcarlo1@unl.edu

Miguel A. Carranza Department of Sociology, University of Nebraska, Lincoln, NE, USA, mcarranza1@unl.edu

Ana Mari Cauce Department of Psychology, Department of American Ethnic Studies, University of Washington, Seattle, WA, USA, cauce@uw.edu

Rand Conger Division of Human Development and Family Studies, Department of Human and Community Development, Department of Psychology, University of California, Davis, Davis, CA, USA, rdconger@ucdavis.edu

Marissa Corona Department of Psychology, University of Washington, Seattle, WA, USA, mcorona@uw.edu

Lisa J. Crockett Department of Psychology, University of Nebraska, Lincoln, NE, USA, ecrockett1@unl.edu

Rick Cruz Department of Psychology, University of Washington, Seattle, WA, USA, cruzr1@uw.edu

Andrew J. Fuligni University of California, Los Angeles, CA, USA, afuligni@ucla.edu

Sandra Graham Department of Education, University of California, Los Angeles, CA 90095-1521, USA, shgraham@ucla.edu

Miriam M. Martinez University of Nebraska, Lincoln, NE, USA, martinez_m4@hotmail.com

Vonnie C. McLoyd Department of Psychology, University of North Carolina, Chapel Hill, NC 27599, USA, vcmcloyd@unc.edu

William M. Sribney Third Way Statistics, White Lake, NY, USA, wsribney@stata.com

William A. Vega Edward R. Roybal Institute on Aging, University of Southern California (USC), Los Angeles, CA 90089-041, USA, williaav@usc.edu

Les B. Whitbeck Department of Sociology, University of Nebraska-Lincoln, Lincoln, NE 68588-0324, USA, lwhitbeck2@unlnotes.unl.edu

Understanding Ethnic/Racial Health Disparities in Youth and Families in the US

Gustavo Carlo, Lisa J. Crockett, Miguel A. Carranza, and Miriam M. Martinez

At first glance, one might not consider motivation to be particularly relevant to understanding health disparities. Motivational processes traditionally focus on affective and cognitive mechanisms that help explain the energy associated with engaging in specific actions (Bandura, 2004). However, health outcomes, including physical and psychological health, have been strongly linked to motivational mechanisms, and many psychological theories address important motivational processes associated with health outcomes (e.g., Deci & Ryan, 1991; Ratelle, Vallerand, Chantal, & Provencher, 2004; Taylor & Brown, 1988; Vallerand & Bissonnette, 1992). One challenge is to apply traditional theories of motivation associated with health outcomes to health disparities. The present volume begins to examine the central role of motivation in health disparities. Although health disparities cut across many demographic and personal dimensions, including age, sex, sexual orientation, ethnicity, race, and SES, the present volume focuses primarily on ethnicity, race, and economic class (though other topics such as gender are briefly discussed).

Some National Trends in Health Disparities

There is ample data on health disparities across many domains of functioning. We begin this chapter by presenting data trends in disparities in selected health topics. This brief overview will provide a broad context for understanding pattern of health disparities among youth and families and the many challenges to addressing them. As we present the data, it is important keep in mind the disproportionately high rates of physical and mental health problems among ethnic minority and low SES populations. These disproportionate rates reflect increased risk factors that contribute to the health problems in these minority populations. Thus, one challenge for social scientists is to identify the multiple causal factors that lead to these high rates of health problems.

G. Carlo (✉)
Department of Psychology, University of Nebraska, Lincoln, NE, USA
e-mail: gcarlo1@unl.edu

G. Carlo et al. (eds.), *Health Disparities in Youth and Families*, Nebraska Symposium on Motivation 57, DOI 10.1007/978-1-4419-7092-3_1,
© Springer Science+Business Media, LLC 2011

1

According to the Census Bureau (2007), the estimated population of the US stands at *298,757,310*, of which approximately *14.7% are Latino, 12.4% African American, 4.3% Asian American, and 0.8% Native American.* Moreover, *the overall mean income per capita is $26,178, and* an estimated *13.3% individuals live below the poverty line.* A disproportionate percentage of those living in poverty are ethnic and racial minorities. As many scholars have noted, one major barrier to better health outcomes is poverty (Addler, Boyce, Chesney, Folkman, & Syme, 1993; Lillie-Blanton & Laveist, 1996). However, poverty is not sufficient to account for health disparities among ethnic minorities. The present volume presents additional factors that should be considered as additional sources of variation in health disparities.

One major indicator of health is infant mortality rates. Figure 1 presents a break down of these rates across ethnicity and race. As can be seen, African Americans (13.63), Puerto Ricans (8.30), and Native Americans (8.06) are all above the national average. In contrast, the groups below the national average include Whites (5.76), Mexican Americans (5.53), Asian Americans (4.89), Central and South Americans (4.68), and Cubans (4.42). Furthermore, the fact that there are wide disparities across these groups and even across ethnic subgroups (e.g., within Latinos), point to the importance of examining these issues both within and across culture groups. In a similar vein, Fig. 2 shows that Native Americans, Hispanics, and African Americans are twice as likely to receive inadequate prenatal care as Non-Hispanic Whites. Thus, not all ethnic minorities are equally at risk on these indicators.

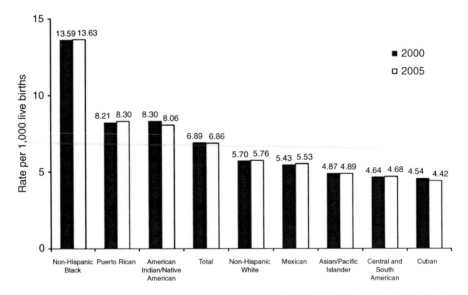

Fig. 1 Infant mortality rates by race and ethnicity: United States, 2000 and 2005. Note: Includes persons of Hispanic and non-Hispanic origin. Source: CDC/NCHS, linked birth infant death data sets, 2000 and 2005

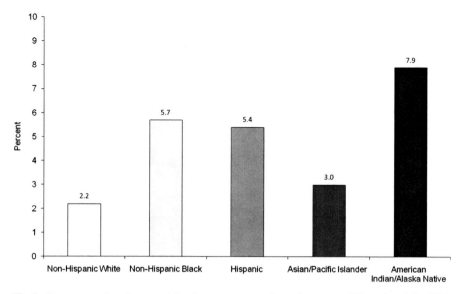

Fig. 2 Percentage of mothers receiving late or no prenatal care by race and Hispanic origin, 2004. Note: Data for 2004 are based on preliminary estimates. Source Hamilton, Martin, Ventura, Sutton, and Menacker (2006)

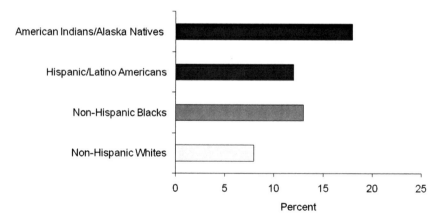

Fig. 3 US deaths due to Diabetes Mellitus in 2002. Source: 1999–2001 National Health Interview Survey and 1999–2000 National Health and Nutrition Examination Survey estimates projected to year 2002. 2002 outpatient database of the Indian Health Service

Other health outcomes show equally complex patterns of disparities. As Fig. 3 shows, Native Americans, Hispanics, and African Americans are at increased deaths from diabetes mellitus. For cigarette smoking, the results demonstrate that Native Americans fare worst compared to other groups (see Fig. 4). With regard to mental and behavioral health indicators such as depression (see Fig. 5), a similar pattern of findings emerges.

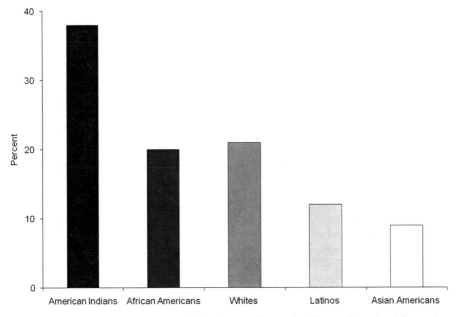

Fig. 4 US current cigarette smoking in 2007. Source: Centers for Disease Control and Prevention (2008)

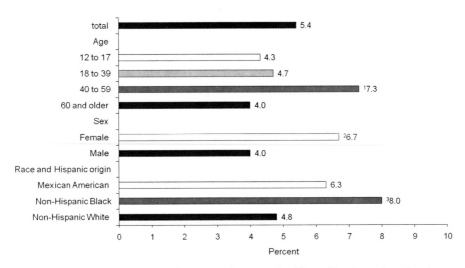

Fig. 5 Percentage of persons 12 years of age and older with depression by demographic characteristics: United States 2005–2006. Note: [1]Significantly different form all other age groups. [2]Significantly different from men. [3]Significantly different from non-Hispanic White persons. Source: CDC/NCHS, National Health and Nutrition Examination Survey

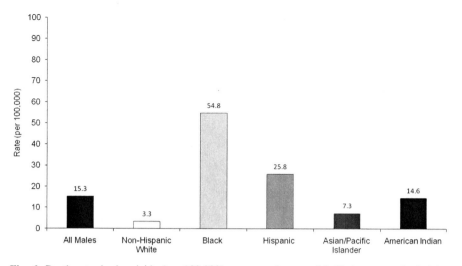

Fig. 6 Death rates by homicide (per 100,000) among males ages 15–19, by race and ethnicity, 2004. Source: Child Trend Databank, 2005

Other health findings reveal even more dramatic differences in rates. One of the most notable findings is the number of homicides per 100,000 among different ethnic/racial groups aged 15–19 years of age. Figure 6 shows that African Americans, Hispanics, Native Americans, and Asian Americans are all more than twice as likely to die from homicide as non-Hispanic Whites. Furthermore, there is huge variability among the ethnic minority groups. The abnormally high rate for young African Americans is striking and reflects a serious health problem in this group. This is an issue that the Children's Defense Fund and other national agencies have sought to address with campaigns such as the *Cradle to Prison Pipeline* program.

What Are Some Factors Associated with Health Disparities?

As noted earlier, among the many factors strongly associated with health disparities, none is more notorious than poverty. As Fig. 7 demonstrates, African Americans, Native Americans, and Latinos are two to three times more likely to live at or below the poverty level. The lack of resources reflective of individuals who live in poverty could lead to deprived family and community environments (e.g., schools with inadequate funding, lack of access to quality medical services). Not surprisingly, figures on educational attainment show patterns consistent with this notion (see Fig. 8). Moreover, Fig. 9 yields evidence that a substantial number of ethnic minorities also lack health insurance. These data suggest that the identification of demographic contextual variables can be one useful avenue for understanding health disparities.

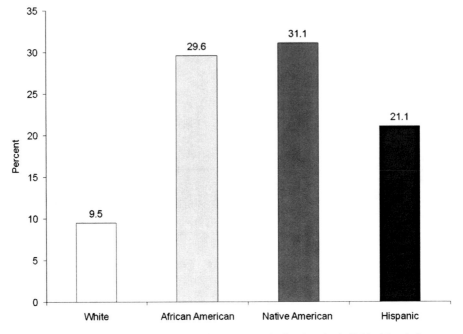

Fig. 7 US rates of poverty in 2006. Note: Percentage calculated at the individual level. Source: US Census Bureau, 2006 American Community Survey

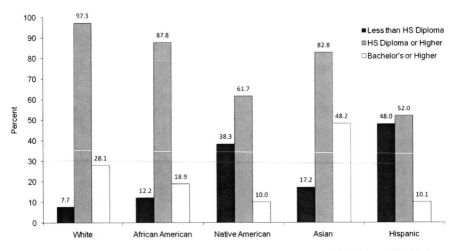

Fig. 8 Educational attainment for the population 25 years and over 2006. Note: HS Diploma includes equivalency. Persons of Hispanic origin might be any race. Source: US Census Bureau, 2006 American Community Survey

However, to understand the root causes of health disparities requires theories and models that integrate personal and contextual level variables. Cultural context and culture socialization theorists suggest that individual and group differences in behavioral and psychological outcomes can be explained by cognitive

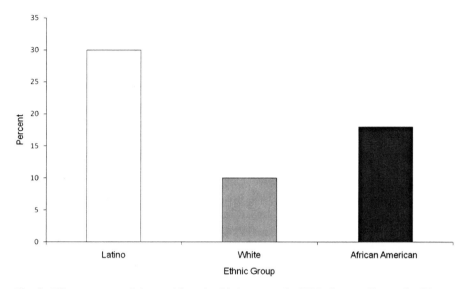

Fig. 9 US percentage of those without health insurance in 2008. Source: Center for Disease Control and Prevention

and affective, as well as social contextual, mechanisms. Thus there is a need for theories that integrate motivational and culture-specific factors into existing models of health behaviors. The chapters in this volume address this need and advance our understanding of specific mechanisms contributing to health disparities.

In the chapter "The Face of the Future: Risk and Resilience in Minority Youth", Anna Marie Cauce and her colleagues begin the book by providing a broad overview of health disparities among African American, Latino, and White youth in the United States. Their chapter illustrates, through research and anecdotes, some of the major challenges facing our ethnic/racial groups today. For these scholars, health disparities begin in the communities and school environments that youth are residing in. These contextual factors have an important cascade of health consequences that operate through socialization (e.g., family and peer processes) and stress-related experiences. Although they outline a number of disheartening rates of violence, mental illness, and substance use disorders, they also offer hope for future generations of ethnic minority youth owing to existing protective factors and the changing face of majority–minority status in our society. As ethnic minorities come to represent the majority of the US population, some health problems associated with minority status should dissipate. Moreover, throughout the chapter, references to the life of President Barack Obama are presented as anecdotal evidence for the promise of future generations of ethnic minority youth.

Although poverty is a prime candidate for explaining health disparities in ethnic/racial groups, the evidence for this link is often difficult to obtain. In the chapter "How Money Matters for Children's Socioemotional Adjustment: Family Processes and Parental Investment", Dr. McLoyd summarizes her research team's attempts to address this gap. In an intervention study of rare sophistication and rigor,

Dr. McLoyd presents provocative data that suggests that providing money to assist families living in poverty does not appear sufficient in leading to positive health changes in these families. This work suggests that the solution to addressing health disparities is not simply a matter of wealth—indeed, there may be personal level factors that need to be simultaneously addressed to better address these issues. To focus on contextual variables without considering how individuals perceive their environment, nor without considering the agentic nature of selecting and modifying the environment, would result in an incomplete account of health disparities.

One excellent example of the integration of context and personal variables is Sandra Graham's provocative evidence that disparities in academic achievement and mental health can be partly explained by the ethnic composition of school populations (see the chapter "School Racial/Ethnic Diversity and Disparities in Mental Health and Academic Outcomes"). In schools with greater diversity, ethnic minority students fare better than in schools with less diversity. Of particular interest is her ability to show that these outcomes are explained in part by attribution mechanisms—ethnic minorities in diverse contexts are more likely to make internal attributions rather than external attributions. Unlike external attributions, internal attributions enhance academic motivation. Attributional style thus demonstrates a cognitive process that appears to impact motivation and account for health disparities. Thus, the combination of context and attributional styles helps to better account for health disparities among ethnic minorities. This research has important implications regarding school district policies that affect school population diversity.

In the chapter "Social Identity, Motivation, and Well Being Among Adolescents from Asian and Latin American Backgrounds", Fuligni and his colleagues approach health disparities by identifying culture-specific variables (i.e., cultural and family identity) that are linked to academic motivation and mental health. Cultural (or ethnic) identity is defined as the extent to which one's self concept is linked to their ethnic group. Family identity refers to a sense of obligation to support, assist and respect authority figures in the family group. Fuligni shows that these constructs are interrelated and relevant in understanding Latino and Asian American youth development. In general, their studies yield evidence that both constructs predict positive adjustment in both ethnic minority groups. Fuligni's findings are consistent with those of other scholars (e.g., Armenta, Knight, Carlo, & Jacobson, in press; Phinney, Jacoby, & Silva, 2007; Umaña-Taylor, Diversi, & Fine, 2002). Although Fuligni notes that cultural and family identity are not sufficient predictors of well being in ethnic minorities, their work yields promising evidence on the relevance of culture-specific variables that can account for health disparities among ethnic minority groups.

The dramatic rates of psychological and behavioral pathology among Native American youth reflect one of the greatest challenges in addressing ethnic group health disparity. There is a long and well documented history of abuse and neglect of this ethnic group in the United States that has undoubtedly resulted in the malaise that is evident today. The research findings regarding the high rates of substance use and mental illness among early adolescents presented by Whitbeck and his associates (see the chapter "The Beginnings of Mental Health Disparities: Emergent

Mental Disorders Among Indigenous Adolescents") are alarming. Utilizing a comprehensive model that includes culture specific variables, as well as person-level and contextual variables, to guide their research and intervention efforts, they summarize what is perhaps the most comprehensive and rigorous research and intervention work to date in this ethnic group. Among the several lessons learned from their work is the emphasis on creating cultural partnerships in the communities in conducting research and providing services as well as a focus on risk and protective factors. They conclude their chapter by listing a set of policy and intervention recommendations to address the numerous health disparities in this often maligned and marginalized population.

Focusing on Latinos, Vega and Sribney conduct a thorough analysis and critique of the various challenges of understanding and addressing health disparities in this ethnic group (see the chapter "Understanding the Hispanic Health Paradox Through a Multi-Generation Lens: A Focus on Behavior Disorders"). One of the major challenges is to understand the so-called, "Hispanic Health Paradox." This refers to the often cited finding that second and later generation Hispanics fare worse across a number of health indicators than first generation (native born) Hispanics. Utilizing trans-generational data, these scholars demonstrate the complexity of addressing health disparities—they show that health problems increase across generations and suggest that such increases are likely genetically based. Based on research from geneticists, Vega and Sribney propose that behavioral health changes that result from immigration to new environments might result in changes in genetic vulnerability in the population. Although much more research is needed, the introduction of biological-based mechanisms into existing theories of health disparities in ethnic/racial groups is a provocative new direction for future researchers. Furthermore, Vega and Sribney remind us of the importance of attending to within-culture variation as well as between-culture variation. For example, their findings yield evidence on gender-specific patterns of health outcomes among Latinos that must be understood as we move forward on addressing health disparities across different ethnic/racial groups.

Summary and Conclusions

To summarize, ethnic and social class disparities are evident across a spectrum of markers of psychological, behavioral, and physical health. Furthermore, the pattern is often complex such that disparities are sometimes found within ethnic/racial groups as well as across those groups. Indeed, it is likely that the causes of health disparities may be different across specific subgroups. Moreover, theoretical models are needed that examine biological, contextual, and person-level variables (including culture-specific variables) to account for health disparities. The scholars in the present volume provide exemplary research that moves us towards more comprehensive and integrative models of health disparities. A brief glance at the work summarized by these scholars yields some common elements of focus for future researchers regarding risk (e.g., poverty, lack of contextual diversity) and protective (e.g., family support, cultural identity) factors yet they also identify aspects (e.g., genetic vulnerabilities) that may be unique to specific ethnic/racial groups.

In addition to employing more integrative and culturally sensitive models of health disparities, future research studies could expand the scope of investigation to include transnational studies of health disparities and the processes contributing to them. They might also consider culture-specific health problems and syndromes such as "nervios" in Latino cultures. Within nations, further attention might be directed to the community contexts in which ethnic minority and low SES families reside, not only urban areas but the much less studied rural areas. Finally, efforts to assess health disparities and the factors contributing to them across cultural and ethnic groups need to attend closely to the issue of measurement equivalence in order to ensure valid cross-group comparisons. We would add that future research on health disparities will need to examine markers of positive health outcomes and well being (e.g., social competence) rather than focusing solely on risk and protective factors associated with health-related problems. We cannot assume that the relative absence of negative pathology and risk equals the presence of health and well being—thus research is needed that includes both positive and negative health outcomes. More attention to positive health indicators will further our understanding of normative, positive health outcomes and lead us away from traditional deficit and pathology-focused models of ethnic minorities. Finally, the scholars in this volume all present findings that have important implications for policy and intervention efforts—the lessons learned from their efforts should be heeded if we are to comprehensively and effectively address the existing health disparities in the US.

Acknowledgements The volume editors would like to acknowledge the valuable contributions and assistance of the numerous people who made this work possible, including Debra Hope, Claudia Price-Decker, Roxane Earnest, Jamie Longwell, Jodi Carter, Kate Duangdao, and the Psychology office student workers. Others who support this work in important ways include Chancellor Harvey Perlman, the NU Foundation, the UNL Latino Research Initiative, and Springer-Verlag Science Publishers (especially Ana Tobias). Special thanks also to the numerous colleagues, conference attendees and students who participated and contributed to the Symposium activities.

References

Addler, N. E., Boyce, W. T., Chesney, M. A., Folkman, S., & Syme, S. L. (1993). Socioeconomic inequalities in health: No easy solution. *Journal of American Medical Association, 269*, 3140–3145.

Armenta, B. E., Knight, G. P., Carlo, G., & Jacobson, R. P. (in press). The relation between ethnic group attachment and prosocial tendencies: The mediating role of ethnically related cultural values. *European Journal of Social Psychology*.

Bandura, A. (2004). Health promotion by social cognitive means. *Health Education & Behavior, 31*(2), 143–164.

Census Bureau U.S. (2007). *Annual population estimates: 2007*. Retrieved May 3, 2010, from http://www.census.gov/popest/estimates.html

Centers for Disease Control and Prevention (2008). Cigarette smoking among adults – United States, 2007. *Morbidity and Mortality Weekly Report*, 57(45):1221–1226.

Deci, E. L., & Ryan, R. M. (1991). A motivational approach to self: Integration in personality. In R. Dienstbier (Ed.), *Nebraska symposium on motivation: Perspectives on motivation* (Vol. 38, pp. 237–288). Lincoln, NE: University of Nebraska Press.

Hamilton, B. E., Martin, J. A., Ventura, S. J., Sutton, P. D., & Menacker, F. (2006). Births: Preliminary data for 2004. *National Vital Statistics Reports, 54*(8). Hyattsville, MD: National Center for Health Statistics.

Lillie-Blanton, M., & Laveist, T. (1996). Race/ethnicity, the social environment, and health. *Social Science and Medicine, 43*(1), 83–91.

Phinney, J., Jacoby, B., & Silva, C. (2007). Positive intergroup attitudes: The role of ethnic identity. *International Journal of Behavioral Development, 31*(5), 478–490.

Ratelle, C., Vallerand, R., Chantal, Y., & Provencher, P. (2004). Cognitive adaptation and mental health: A motivational analysis. *European Journal of Social Psychology, 34*(4), 459–476.

Taylor, S. E., & Brown, J. D. (1988). Illusion and well-being: A social psychological perspective on mental health. *Psychological Bulletin, 103*, 193–210.

Umaña-Taylor, A., Diversi, M., & Fine, M. (2002). Ethnic identity and self-esteem of Latino adolescents: Distinctions among the Latino populations. *Journal of Adolescent Research, 17*(3), 303–327.

Vallerand, R. J., & Bissonnette, R. (1992). Intrinsic, extrinsic, and motivational styles as predictors of behavior: A prospective study. *Journal of Personality, 60*, 599–620.

The Face of the Future:
Risk and Resilience in Minority Youth

Ana Mari Cauce, Rick Cruz, Marissa Corona, and Rand Conger

About a decade ago, as we moved into a new millennium, demographers and jour-nalists galore noted that the "look" of America was changing. But, not a one of them would have predicted that this new look would be seen so soon in the face of our nation's President.

The Presidency of a bi-racial Black man, part of an extended family that he described as a "mini-United Nations" and that includes Kansonians, Southeast Asians, Ethiopians, Christians, and Muslims, was not easily predictable, especially by those in the baby-boom or pre-boomer generations. Yet, from a demographic per-spective, there is nothing anomalous about his background. Not only does President Obama's multiracial background foreshadow the look of the future, it is what present day America already looks like for those of us who work with youth. For example, Fig. 1 shows the racial and ethnic distribution of the US population under 18 based on present census data and on projections for 2020. Fueled by immigration and larger family sizes, racial and ethnic minorities already account for more than 40% of today's youth. In a quarter of US counties, such youth are already a majority, and no longer a minority (Roberts, 2008).

Is this majority–minority future something to look forward to, or something to worry about and fear? This chapter will address this question by first focusing on adolescence as a critical life stage, especially for minority youth. We first examine behavioral, educational, and related indices of well-being among this age group and then move on to review the literature on two key factors that affect youth development—the neighborhood/school context, and the family context and parent-ing styles. These factors can serve to increase the risk for negative developmental outcomes or to mitigate the risk and lead to resilience. They were chosen because they serve as good examples of factors at different points along the ecological con-tinuum, with neighborhood and school more distal influences, and parenting acting as a more proximal influence. Throughout we focus on African-Americans and Latinos, the two minority groups that our research teams have worked with most

A.M. Cauce (✉)
Department of Psychology, Department of American Ethnic Studies, University of Washington, Seattle, WA, USA
e-mail: cauce@uw.edu

G. Carlo et al. (eds.), *Health Disparities in Youth and Families*, Nebraska Symposium on Motivation 57, DOI 10.1007/978-1-4419-7092-3_2, © Springer Science+Business Media, LLC 2011

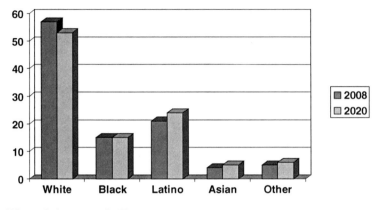

Fig. 1 US population—ages 0–17

closely, and groups where the data base is strongest, albeit still more limited than desirable. At various points, we will use the Obama story, which has been told and re-told so often these last few years, to illustrate how these general processes might play out in the life of a specific individual and family. While science necessarily focuses on understanding general principles, it is applying these principles in order to enhance the lives of individuals that ultimately is of interest to us.

Adolescence as a Critical Life Stage

Adolescence holds a special role in virtually all cultures as a time of transition between childhood and adulthood. It is time of rapid physical and cognitive growth, second only to the first 2 years of life in the amount of change that takes place in a short time span. This, in turn, necessitates adjustments and realignments within the family, as young people are granted a new status in relationships with others in their social world (see Feldman & Elliott, 1990 for a good overview of this life stage).

Adolescence brings new freedoms. Some of these freedoms are small, like moving between classrooms, when previously it was the teachers who moved around. Some are major, like beginning to date, obtaining a driver's license, or a car of one's own. The unique combination of youthful vigor and maturing sensibilities and passions can make this a time of incredible achievements; adolescents have started companies, written symphonies, painted masterpieces, and led armies. But, this troika of physical, cognitive, and social changes, which do not always happen in the preferred order, also lead to heightened vulnerability for youth, as physical maturation is often attained well before brain development has completed (Dahl, 2004). Particularly noteworthy is the slower development of the brain's frontal lobes, which continue to develop through the mid-twenties, especially for boys. Given the rapid and asynchronous growth in these years, it is not altogether surprising that adolescence is also marked by impulsive behavior and imprudent risk-taking. Hence adolescents and their families too often deal with the negative consequences that come from car accidents, unwanted pregnancy, sexually transmitted diseases, and alcohol and drug use.

In light of this vulnerability, adolescence, at least in its ideal form, is a relatively protected time of exploration, where youths can try on adult roles without fully taking on adult responsibilities. However, the ideal may be much more typical of majority youth, especially those from middle-class or affluent backgrounds. This protected period may actually be getting longer for such youth, as they stay in school for extended periods of time. But it may not exist at all for others whose families do not have the wherewithal or resources to protect them from adult responsibilities or the consequences of taking them on so early in life (Burton, Obeidallah, & Allison, 1996).

Foreshadowing the Future: Mental Health, Well-Being, and Educational Outcomes for African-American and Latino Youths

Assessing the mental health status and well-being of Latino and African-American youth is neither easy nor straightforward. The gold standard for gauging the prevalence of mental health disorders in a population is established through epidemiological studies that assess psychiatric disorders as measured by the Diagnostic Statistical Manual, which at present is in its fourth edition (APA, 2000). Over the last decade there have been various large, population-based epidemiological studies conducted with Latinos and/or African-Americans (Takeuchi, Alegria, Jackson, & Williams, 2007). Unfortunately, these have focused only on adults and there are no equivalent studies on children and youth. More recently, the National Comorbidity Survey-Replication (NCS-R: Kessler & Merkikangas, 2004; Kessler et al., 2009) did include a multi-ethnic adolescent sample, but results by race and ethnicity are not yet available.

Fortunately, a number of other national data bases that include indicators of mental health and problem behaviors provide us with a reasonably good indication of how African-American and Latino youth fare compared to their White counterparts. The most comprehensive of these is the U.S. Centers for Disease Control and Prevention (CDC) *Youth Risk Behavior Surveillance* System (CDC, 2007) which includes a national school-based survey which monitors health-risk behaviors among students in grades 9–12.

Figure 2 shows survey responses to questions about participation in problem or deviant behavior, including violence (e.g. been in a physical fight one of more times during the last 12 months, carried a weapon at least 1 day in last 30 days), risky sexual behavior that could lead to pregnancy and sexually transmitted diseases, including HIV infection (e.g. sexually active in last 3 months, had sexual intercourse with four or more persons during life), and emotional distress (e.g. attempted suicide in last 12 months, sadness or hopelessness which prevented usual activities). In general, these results suggest that African-American and Latino youth are more

Fig. 2 Selected risk or
problem behaviour in high
school students (2007)

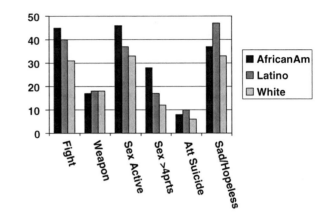

likely to participate in risk behavior related to violence and sexual risk than their
White counterparts. They are also more apt to show signs of emotional distress.

Another national data set that examines adolescent health across ethnic groups is
the National Survey of Children's Health which interviewed parents by telephone.
An analysis of this data (Fox et al., 2007) also provides some reason to be concerned
about African-American and Latino youth. Figure 3 shows health disparities for
adolescents ages 12 through 17 and indicates that African-American, and Latino
youth fare considerably less well than White youth on key health-relevant indicators,
including being overweight or at risk of overweight and in poor health. They also
exercise less than is optimal.

Fig. 3 Health
status—National Alliance to
Advance Adolescent Health

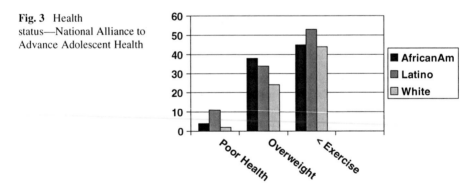

These results are reinforced by results from the National Health and Nutrition
Examination Survey (NHANES) which indicate that African-American female
youth have higher overweight rates than White and Mexican American females.,
Among males, Mexican Americans are significantly more likely to be overweight
than White and African-American youths (Ogden et al., 2006). In addition, Latino
youths have been found to engage is less exercise than either their African-American

or White counterparts (Fox et al., 2007). However, it is important to recognize the limited access to resources among such groups. For instance, low income minority adolescents report having reduced access to recreational facilities in their neighborhoods, which leads to less physical activity and, in turn, increased levels of overweight status (Gordon-Larsen, Nelson, Page, & Popkin, 2006). Individuals living in low income neighborhoods also have less access to the types of grocery stores that allow them to buy healthy, high nutrition food for themselves and their families (Morland, Wing, Roux, & Poole, 2002).

One further area of concern is the higher rate of adolescent pregnancy and birth for Latino youth. As seen in Fig. 4, by the age of 15 African-American and Latino youth are already more than twice as likely to give birth than White youth, with that trend continuing into the later teens (Martin et al., 2009).

An additional source of information about the state of adolescents are the reports and data briefs issued by *Child Trends*, especially those briefs released as part of their *Current Population Series* in 2007. These draw upon population surveys administered by the CDC, National Center for Health Statistics, or National Center for Education Statistics. Figure 5, which is based on this data, shows the percentage of African-American, Latino, and White youths, aged 16–19, who are neither engaged in paid work or in school. The fact that African-American and Latino youth

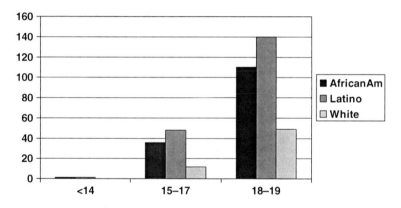

Fig. 4 Adolescent births per 1,000 (2006)

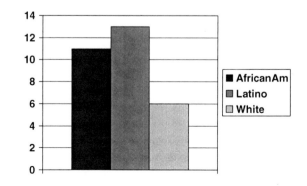

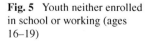

Fig. 5 Youth neither enrolled in school or working (ages 16–19)

are about twice as likely as their White counterparts to be disengaged from conventional society by the time they are entering adulthood is especially disturbing (Wirt et al., 2006).

In sum, while the research available on mental health and well-being amongst minority youth is not as comprehensive as desirable, results are fairly consistent in suggesting that African-American and Latino adolescents are not faring as well as their White counterparts. Whether looking at indicators of emotional distress, risk or problem behaviors, physical health, teen births, or school and job involvement, there is reason for concern.

As shown in Fig. 6, by the time African-American and Latino youth are 25–29, the negative risk, health, and problem behavior just documented has solidified into even more negative outcomes with lifelong consequences. By early adulthood, compared to Whites, more African-Americans and Latinos have failed to complete high school, and a much higher percentage of males are in state, federal or local jails (Brown, Moore, & Bzostek, 2004).

Fig. 6 Young adult outcomes—child trends

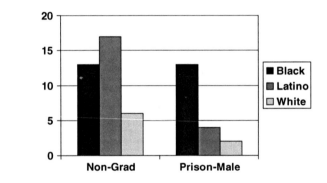

Many of the negative indicators just reviewed are highly correlated to factors that transcend race and ethnicity, such a low socioeconomic status which is nested within race/ethnicity. Nonetheless, based on these data, it is hard to escape the conclusion that, to the degree that the past predicts the future, a future that is more Black and Brown is not necessarily an America that will be healthier or more nationally competitive.

Despite what these indicators predict for our nation's youth of color, President Barrack Obama represents their potential. As recounted in his autobiography, *Dreams of My Father* (Obama, 1995), Obama was born to a young mother and raised apart from his father. His adolescent years were not easy and his search for identity difficult and marked by at least moments of considerable emotional distress and some experimental drug use. At various points in his life, he would not have scored especially high on an adolescent well-being index and he would have showed up on the positive side of some problem behavior measures. In the face of risks aplenty, he overcame adversity to achieve at the highest level. Whether his presidency comes to be known as a successful one or not, there is no question that he, a graduate of Columbia and Harvard universities, a renowned author, politician and world leader, a Nobel prize winner, and by all accounts a loving husband and father, is a success. If his is the face of the future, we have much to look forward to.

We refer to President Obama, and others who, like him, have succeeded in the face of multiple risks in their life as "resilient." This descriptor may bring to mind a bo-bo doll, that always bounces back despite a barrage of punches or kicks. However, research conducted in the last several decades suggests that it is best to think about resilience, not as a characteristic of the individual, but rather as both a process, that evolves over time, and as a product of one's environment, including the people, institutions, or practices in it that can mitigate the effects of risks upon the individual (Masten & Obradović, 2006; Luthar, Cicchetti, & Becker, 2000).

Ecological theory, whether in its original form (Bronfenbrenner, 1979), or as adapted to more specifically encompass minority youth (Garcia Coll et al., 1996) predicts that people are affected by the places and contexts in which they spend time. Those people and contexts closer, or more proximal, to youths, such as their families, have the greatest influence on their lives. But, more distal environments, such as the school or neighborhood environment, can also have powerful effects. These effects can be direct, as when a neighborhood with a high concentration of drug activities makes it easier to obtain drugs or when a neighborhood with lots of parks and recreational facilities makes it easier for children to exercise. Distal environments can also affect a youth directly through their effects on proximal environments. For example, if a parent's workplace adopts policies that make it easier for them to take time off for family issues, it will facilitate good parenting.

The Neighborhood Context for African-American and Latino Youth

With the greater autonomy and freedom accorded to adolescents, they spend increasingly large amounts of time outside the home, and in their neighborhoods. As such, in recent years, there has been growing interest among researchers in how neighborhoods affect those residing in them, especially adolescents and their families (Brooks-Gunn, Duncan, Klebanov, & Sealand, 1993; Haynie, Silver, & Teasdale, 2006; Roosa et al., 2009).

There is little question but that most parents want their children to grow up in what are considered "good" neighborhoods with high quality schools, successful and pro-social neighbors, and safe surroundings. Various attempts have been made to assess neighborhoods over the last decade on the diversity of characteristics that matter to families (Israel et al., 2006). Despite its rather narrow focus, one of the most straightforward and widely used ways to categorize neighborhoods is by poverty level. From this perspective, neighborhoods where more than 40% of the residents are at or below the federal poverty level are called "extremely poor", those where 20% or more of the residents are below the poverty level are called "poor" or "high poverty", and those where less than 20% of the residents are below the poverty level are considered "non-poor" (Jargowsky & Bane, 1991). Among non-poor neighborhoods, those where less than 10% are poor are called "low poverty" and those where less than 3% are poor are considered "affluent" (Timberlake & Michael, 2006).

As we began this decade, less than 15% of extremely poor neighborhoods were primarily White, while two thirds of them were primarily African-American or Latino (Jargowsky, 1997). Moreover, almost half of all African-Americans (48%) and Latinos (43%) live in neighborhoods where their own ethnicity made up the majority of the population (e.g. 48% of African-Americans live in majority African-American communities). Putting these facts together, it becomes clear that many African-American and Latino youths are growing up in neighborhoods where they are both economically and ethnically isolated.

A recent analysis of trends in the ethnic and socioeconomic composition of neighborhoods during the 1990s found that more than 80% of White children were born into non-poor or low poverty neighborhoods. In contrast, this was the case for less than half of African-American or Latino children. On the other end of the continuum, White children were almost four times as likely as African-American children and ten times as likely as Latino children to be born into an affluent neighborhood (Timberlake, 2006).

African-American and Latino children born into high poverty neighborhoods were also more likely to remain in high poverty neighborhoods, or to move into extremely poor neighborhoods, than similar White youth. African-Americans born in high poverty neighborhoods typically spend about 70% of their childhoods there, with more than a third of that time in an extremely poor neighborhood. By contrast, White children born in high poverty neighborhoods spend less than 10% of their time in neighborhoods characterized by extreme poverty (Timberlake, 2006). Therefore, the neighborhood advantage enjoyed by White youth at birth is magnified if one assumes that the effects of neighborhood accumulate over time.

There is substantial room for debate about the magnitude and range of effects of growing up in poor neighborhoods. But, while some studies have found much larger and wide-ranging effects than others, the evidence clearly shows that youth who grow up in high poverty neighborhoods are less likely to complete high school, and more likely to become teenage parents (Brooks-Gunn, Duncan, & Aber, 1997; Crane, 1991). Some studies have suggested that it is the absence of affluence or wealth that leads to poorer outcomes for youth, rather than the presence of poverty per se (Wen, Browning, & Cagney, 2003). Others researchers have suggested that it is the nexus between poverty and ethnicity which traps so many minorities in *ghettos* or *barrios* that may be most harmful. In his book, *Poverty and Place: Neighborhoods, Barrios and the American City* (1997), economist Paul Jargowsky argues that it is not any one, but rather a multiplicity of factors, that leads to more negative outcomes for youth growing up in these poor, largely minority, neighborhoods. He argues that chief among them is the culture in poor neighborhoods that places more importance on short-term goals over long-term ones, the dearth of positive role models for youth in poor neighborhoods, and the way living in poor neighborhoods isolate youths and families from connections to more affluent individuals and organizations that can lead to future job opportunities.

A recent report of the Pew Foundation's Economic Mobility Project (Sharkey, 2009) found that growing up in a poor neighborhood increases a youth's chances of downward economic mobility by a staggering 52%. Indeed, the study concludes that childhood neighborhood poverty accounts for a bigger share of the black-white gap in downward mobility than parent's education, occupation, or labor force participation. In this way, the effects of living in a high poverty neighborhood reverberates into a child's future.

In addition to the social and psychological effects that may stem from coming of age in a poor neighborhood, these neighborhoods, and the schools within them, pose real physical dangers for youth, turning them not only into places of potential failure, but ones of fear. Some have gone so far as to compare some inner-city neighborhoods to war zones because of their high crime rates. These crimes are often perpetrated on youth by other youths, whether alone or in gangs (Garbarino, 2001).

Most of us know that youth, between the ages of 15 and 25, commit a disproportionate amount of crime, especially violent crime (Loeber & Farrington, 2001). Fewer are aware that youth are also more apt to be the victims of crime, especially when the offender is another youth. About two-thirds of all crimes experienced by those under 18 are committed by other youths, and over 90% of all sexual crimes committed by youths have other youths as victims (Office of Justice Programs, 2009). More generally, regardless of the age of the perpetrator, adolescents are twice as likely to be victimized as the national average, with 12–15 year olds the age group most apt to be victimized (Perkins, 1997).

The most common form of crime experienced by adolescents is property crime—having a bike stolen, backpack taken, or camera or I-Pod snatched. When compared to Whites, African-American youth were somewhat more apt than youth of other ethnicities to experience this type of crime, although there is no statistical difference between African-Americans and Latinos (Finklehor & Ormrod, 2000). However, the disparities in rates of victimization become more pronounced when violent crimes, especially serious violent crimes, are examined.

When rates of victimization by serious violent crimes, including homicide, rape, and aggravated assault, were examined, they were about twice (13.5 per 1,000) as high for African-Americans than for their White counterparts (6.5 per 1,000; Bureau of Justice Statistics, 2006). Moreover, while less than a third (31%) of non-fatal crimes were classified as "serious" among White youth, serious, they represented 40% of similar crimes for Latinos and 48% of those crimes for Africans (Bureau of Justice Statistics, 2007).

Figure 7 shows youth mortality rates for African-American, Latino, and White males. Race and ethnic disparities are most marked when homicide is examined, with African-Americans six times more likely to be victims of homicide than Whites, and Latinos murdered about three times more often (Aguirre, Turner, & Aguirre, 2008). In addition to being more often directly victimized, African-American and Latino youth living in high poverty neighborhoods are more apt to experience secondary exposure to violence, as defined by witnessing it. Higher rates of exposure to secondary violence are also more common in neighborhoods with higher concentrations of immigrant youths (Gibson, Morris, & Beaver, 2009).

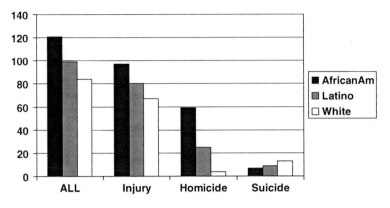

Fig. 7 Male youth mortality rate (15–19)

The type of violence we have just described does not just happen in housing projects or back alleyways. One of the places within their neighborhoods where youth experience violence and victimization is their school. African-American and Latino youth clearly report being more afraid of violence and victimization inside their school than do White youth. In the mid-90 s more than 20% of African-American and Latino youth reported that they felt afraid at school, or on the way to school, compared to 8% of their White counterparts. Although rates of victimization, and hence fear, fell considerably over the next decade, in 2005 African-American and Latino youth continued to feel fear in school at almost twice the rate of others (6–7%) of African-American and Latino youths reported fear, compared to 3–4% of Whites (National Center for Education Statistics, 2009).

African-American and Latino youth are also more likely to report that gangs were present in their school. More than a third of Latino youths, aged 12–18, reported that their schools had gangs, regardless of whether they attended suburban (34.6%) or urban (42.6%) schools. More than a quarter of African-American youths in suburban schools (28.3%) and almost a third of those in urban schools (32.8%) reported the presence of gangs. By comparison less than a fifth of White youth reported the presence of gangs in their school, whether urban (19.8%) or suburban (13.8%) (National Center for Education Statistics, 2009).

In sum, African-American and Latino youths typically grow up in very different neighborhoods than do White youths. These neighborhoods, and the schools within them, have higher concentrations of poverty and expose youth to higher rates of violence, both directly and indirectly. There is no way to downplay the potential risk that African-American and Latino youth face in too many of their neighborhoods and schools. The adverse relationship between negative neighborhood and school characteristics and adolescent's school success, and aggressive behavior, for example, has been found even after controlling for socioeconomic status more generally (Meyers & Miller, 2004). These effects are not only contemporaneous, they reach far into the future.

However it is precisely because of the high density of minorities living in high poverty, high crime neighborhoods, that institutions within minority communities are also more apt to offer services and activities directly geared to their needs. For example, schools with high concentrations of Latino students are more apt to have bilingual teachers, and there is a higher chance of finding ESL (English as a second language) services in these neighborhoods or *barrios* (Katz, 1999; Patthey-Chavez, 1993). Neighborhoods with a high concentration of Latinos are more apt to have grocery stores with Latino foods, and to have bilingual clerks at supermarkets or banks. In a similar vein, neighborhoods with high concentrations of African-Americans are more apt to find barbershops or beauty shops with hairstylists used to working with thick, curly hair, and retail stores carrying products aimed at African-Americans. The dangers of crime are all too apparent and quite real, but there are other risks involved in being in a neighborhood or school where one is in the minority, or the "only" (see Mengesha, 2009 for a description of being "the only Black student" in a college setting). A comprehensive study of neighborhood mobility and selection (Sampson & Sharkey, 2008) found that African-Americans in Chicago ended up in ethnically isolated neighborhoods in large part, due to the fact that others tended to exit neighborhoods with growing concentrations of Blacks. But, it was also the case that African-American families, even those with the means to make the choice, felt they could either live in a more affluent (White) neighborhood or in a more hospitable and racially diverse neighborhood, what the authors called "a not unreasonable calculus given the grim history of race relations in Chicago" (p. 26). Indeed, while it is typical for White youth to live in a low poverty or affluent neighborhood that is also culturally consonant and responsive, this is an extremely rare experience for African-American or Latino youth. Regardless of exactly how the incident ensued or what it says about racial profiling, the recent arrest of Professor Henry Louis Gates (Editors, New York Times, 2009) in his own house, in an affluent Cambridge neighborhood near Harvard University, was viewed by many as one more reminder that African-Americans or Latinos are only *guests* in such neighborhoods. Too often they are viewed by their White neighbors as at best simply outsiders, and, more often, with suspicion and fear.

Barack Obama was raised in a very unique setting, or set of settings. He spent his primary school years living in Indonesia, attending public and private schools there, followed by grades five to high school living in Hawaii and attending Ponahou School, both of which are noteworthy as truly multicultural environments. While African-Americans are minorities in Hawaii, so are Whites. In describing his experiences there Obama wrote, "The opportunity that Hawaii offered—to experience a variety of cultures in a climate of mutual respect—became an integral part of my world view, and a basis for the values that I hold most dear" (Charlton, 2007). This opportunity most likely also played a role in his pathway of resilience. But, as we have just illustrated with statistics and examples, we have a long way to go as a society before more African-American and Latino youth have a similar opportunity to grow up in non-poverty, safe, neighborhoods and school where they also feel a strong sense of respect and belonging.

Parenting in African-American and Latino Adolescents: Risk and Protection

No matter how involved youths may be in their neighborhoods and school, their parents typically stand a step closer to them, exerting both a stronger direct influence, and potentially mediating the effects of the neighborhood on their children. When researchers and policy makers first turned their attention to the unique aspects of parenting minority youth, their assessments were generally negative. Minority families, especially female-headed African-American families, were described as a "tangle of pathology" that either manufactured or promoted cultural disadvantage (U.S. Department of Labor, 1965). The language of professional researchers may have been less inflammatory, but often their descriptions also led one to conclude that minority families were the cause of their children's ills. Their descriptions of minority parenting typically portrayed them as overly authoritarian, intrusive, and punitive, or disengaged and absent (see Cauce, Coronado, & Watson, 1998, for a description of models used to assess minority families).

Recent comprehensive examinations of minority families have resulted in a much more nuanced portrait of them. These studies highlight the fact that African-American and Latino mothers and fathers often parent under conditions that can only be described as highly stressful. They typically face greater challenges to their parenting abilities than most White parents because of the high risk conditions that surround their children, including the more violent neighborhood and school environments we just described. In addition to facing greater challenges, they often have fewer resources to draw-upon, given their higher rates of poverty, with African-American and Latino youths are two to three times as likely to grow up in poverty (Proctor & Dalakar, 2002). These higher rates of poverty put children at risk for a host of negative outcomes, including poorer physical and mental health, school achievement, and involvement with violent or victimizing peer groups (Bradley & Corwyn, 2002; Conger, Ge, Elder, Lorenz & Simmons, 1994; Luthar, 1999; McLoyd, 1998). Poverty also affects parenting. McLoyd and colleagues have written extensively about the challenges faced by parents with very limited financial resources and how that can disrupt parenting (Ceballo & McLoyd, 2002; Huston et al., 2001; Mistry, Vandewater, Huston, & McLoyd, 2002). To state it bluntly, parenting while poor can readily turn into poor parenting.

The family stress model developed by Conger and colleagues (Conger, Conger, Elder, Lorenz, & Simons, 1994; Conger, Rueter, & Conger, 2000) describes how poverty puts a great deal of stress on the individual parent, and in two-parent families, on the mariial relationships. This stress leads to family dysfunction and distress and to parenting practices and parenting that can be at once overly harsh, and insufficiently warm and involved. Parents who experience high levels of stress are more likely to be punitive, react irritably with their children, and to exert discipline in a manner that is more inconsistent (Conger et al., 2000; Deater-Deckard, Dodge, Bates, & Pettit, 1996; McLoyd & Smith, 2002). In turn, there is good evidence that this type of inconsistent parenting can contribute to adolescent conduct problems and lowered academic achievement (Loeber, Stouthamer-Loeber, 1996; Smith & Thornberry, 1995; Thornberry & Krohn, 2003).

Yet, despite the stress so often experienced by African-American and Latino families, especially those in high risk neighborhoods, not all parenting is disrupted.

There is much evidence that warm and involved parenting can serve as a source of protection for adolescents. Minority adolescents generally do better when their parents are warm and use firm, even strict, disciplinary practices. This type of positive parenting can help to protect youth from the negative influences they are exposed to in poor neighborhoods and schools (Brody et al., 2001; Duncan & Raudenbush, 2002; Loukas, Prelow, Suizzo, & Allulua, 2008; O'Donnell, Schwab-Stone, & Muyeed, 2002). While much of this research has been conducted with African-American families, research focusing specifically on Latino families has likewise found that warm, involved parenting can lead to more positive developmental outcomes in their children, even in high risk circumstances (Gandara, 1995; Gonzalez & Padilla, 1997; Hernandez, 1993). For example, family support has been found to moderate the negative effects of acculturative stress on Latino youth (Hovey & King, 1996; Rueschenberg & Buriel, 1989; Sabogal, Marin, Otero-Sabogal, Marin, & Perez-Stable, 1987).

Moreover, some forms of parenting that, on first blush, may appear less than optimal, may work well within these ecological niches. Various studies have suggested that, in part due to the higher risk environments they typically live in, parenting styles that are stricter or more high-control may be adaptive in raising African-American and Latino adolescents so long as the high levels of control are leavened with high warmth and affection (Cauce et al., 1996; McLoyd, Cauce, Takeuchi, & Wilson, 2000; Pittman & Chase-Landsdale, 2001).

More specifically, parental monitoring, defined by parents' knowledge of their children's friends, activities, and whereabouts, appears to play an especially important role in protecting adolescents from harm, and ensuring their positive developmental outcomes. Research with both African-American and Latino families suggests that parental monitoring may be instrumental in shielding adolescents from the anti-social, deviant peer groups found more often in poor neighborhoods and schools (Brody et al., 2001; Gonzales, Cauce, & Mason, 1996; Quane & Rankin, 1998; Rankin & Quane, 2002). Thus, accumulating empirical evidence shows that parenting is both shaped by the social environments that surround families, and in turn, that parenting shapes adolescent behavior. The complex interaction and interplay between these factors is most vividly captured in qualitative studies. In Robin Jarrett's (1997, 1999) ethnographic analyses, she has described the work of African-American parents in high risk neighborhoods as "bridging"; it is their role to provide their children a bridge away from the antisocial values they are exposed to and towards more pro-social, conventional lifestyles and values. Some of what has been described as intrusive, harsh behavior or over-protective parenting, Jarrett describes as parental attempts to shield their children from a street culture that has been described as "predatory". Cauce, Gonzales, Mason and colleagues (Cauce et al., 1996; Mason, Cauce, & Gonzales, 1997; Mason, Cauce, Gonzales, & Hiraga, 1994; Mason, Cauce, Gonzales, & Hiraga, 1996) have likewise described the very real quandary that African-Americans can feel when, on the one hand, they want to support and encourage their teenager's autonomy, but, on the other, want to protect them from the dangers that exist in high risk neighborhoods and schools.

An ethnographic study of Puerto Rican and Mexican American adolescent girls and their mothers led to similar observations. Foremost amongst mother's concerns was fear about their children's exposure to community violence and drug use. In order to counteract these dangers, they paid careful attention to their contacts outside the family, set strict family rules for behavior outside the homes, and involved other family members in the supervision of their daughters (Villarruel, 1998).

It is not surprising that the protective parenting strategies developed by African-American and Latino parents are so similar given the similarities in the risks they face. In this vein, it is important to note that while overly harsh and punitive parenting has been found to lead to poor adolescent outcomes and to magnify risk, what is "optimally" and what is "overly" harsh or strict may vary by context and ethnicity. Numerous studies have found that perhaps overly strict parenting, from a White perspective, might not only be protective, but African-American and Latino youths may interpret the strictness as a sign of their parents love and concern (Dixon, Graber, & Brooks-Gunn, 2008; Mason, Walker-Barnes, Tu, Simons, & Martinez-Arrue, 2004; Parke, 2004).

It is not easy to describe with any accuracy or authority the type of parenting that Barack Obama received, especially given the number of different "primary" caretakers in his life. He lived for a time with his mother and Indonesian stepfather, for a while with his grandparents with a long-distance mother, and for a time with all three. But, extrapolating from his accounts, one could certainly conclude that his family life was characterized by a great deal of warmth and caring, and that when a firm hand was needed, it was there—whether in the form of grandmother, grandfather, or mother. The absence of his father loomed large, and most likely exacerbated the difficulties he had when struggling for ethnic identity. But, all in all, he seems to have mostly experienced the type of positive parenting that leads to desirable outcomes.

Toward a Majority–Minority Future

In this chapter, we have attempted to provide an overview of some of the most salient risks faced by African-American and Latino youth, and also of some of the sources of stress and protection they might experience. In doing so, the view we have provided is a high level one, largely glossing over some of the very real differences between African-Americans and Latinos, as well as the huge diversity within African-American and Latino subgroups. Anyone working directly with youth, whether as a practitioner or researcher, should proceed with care in making generalizations to their specific context and population.

While some general trends can be readily discerned from a review of the literature in this area, there is still a great need for longitudinal research, with good measurement of both the characteristics of minority youth and their families, and of the neighborhoods they live in and schools they attend. While there is much to suggest that risk and resilience accumulates and/or plays out over time, too much of the research is cross-sectional, especially when African American or Latino youth are the subjects of study.

We also know very little about the advantages or risks faced by these youths when they do live in, or attend, more affluent schools. Indeed, it has begun almost common for affluent primary and secondary schools to reach out to poor, but talented, African American and Latino youth, in part, to provide them better educational and social opportunities, and in part, to enrich and diversity the experiences of the affluent White majority student body. But, there has been little long-term follow-up examining how these social experiments impact the social, emotional, and educational outcomes of the youth who experience such dissonance between what they see and experience in their home/neighborhood and school environments. Such studies may help identify what cultural scaffolding may lead to optimal briding between these environments.

In summary, it seems quite clear that any analysis of the social context surrounding African-American and Latino youth will show that, as a group, they start their lives at a disadvantage compared to their White counterparts. They are more likely to be poor, more likely to live in neighborhoods marked by disorganization and violence, and more likely to attend poor quality, potentially violent schools. The same pressures these forces exert on adolescents also create stress for the family, and can disrupt parenting. When parenting is disrupted, environmental risk is magnified for adolescents.

Given the conditions they grow up in, it is no wonder that, on average, African-American and Latino youth often have developmental outcomes that are less than positive. Indeed, for those youth where all of these factors come together, especially in their most negative form, it is hard to imagine positive, or resilient, outcomes. Someone cannot pull themselves up with their bootstraps unless they, at least, have boots.

Fortunately, for many youths there is just enough positive to offset the risk. For example, when parents are able to provide their children with firm and involved parenting, environmental risks can be somewhat mitigated. And, it would be a mistake to believe that even in the worse schools or neighborhoods there are not pockets of protection. Some youth manage to access them, even against the odds.

In order to make abstract points more tangible, we have drawn from Obama's biography, albeit fairly lightly. Obama's writings suggest that while he faced some risks, similar to those of other African-American or Latino youths, he also benefitted from a great deal of protection. Such protection came for him in the form of grandparents providing emotional stability and consistent parenting and a highly educated mother who instilled in him a love of knowledge and passion for learning. He grew up in a safe, middle-class neighborhood, and attended an academically rigorous school. Both of these were located within an extremely multicultural context, which is especially rare in the mainland United States.

Obama's trajectory is surely not a roadmap that the typical African-American or Latino youth, or their parents, can use to plot out a successful path. Still, it does provide a very visible example of just how much is possible. There is no one formula, or magic bullet, to ensure positive outcomes for youth of color, especially the many who experience multiple risks to their well-being. To make that possibility a reality for more of our youth will take the efforts not just of their parents, but of all of us.

References

Aguirre, A., Turner, J. H., & Aguirre, A., Jr. (2008). *American ethnicity: The dynamics and consequences of discrimination*. New York: McGraw-Hill.

American Psychiatric Association. (2000). *Diagnostic and statistical manual of mental disorders DSM-IV-TR* (4th edn). Washington, DC: Author.

Bradley, R. H., & Corwyn, R. F. (2002). Socioeconomic status and child development. *Annual Review of Psychology, 53*, 371–399.

Brody, G. H., Ge, X., Conger, R., Gibbons, F. X., Murry, V. M., Gerrard, M., et al. (2001). The influence of neighborhood disadvantage, collective socialization, and parenting on African American children's affiliation with deviant peers. *Child Development, 72*, 1231–1246.

Bronfenbrenner, U. (1979). *The ecology of human development: Experiments by nature and design*. Cambridge: Harvard University Press.

Brooks-Gunn, J., Duncan, G. J., & Aber, J. L. (1997). *Neighborhood poverty: Context and consequences for children*. New York: Russell Sage.

Brooks-Gunn, J., Duncan, G. J., Klebanov, P. K., & Sealand, N. (1993). Do neighbourhood influence child and adolescent development? *American Journal of Sociology, 99*(2), 353–395.

Brown, B. V., Moore, K. A., & Bzostek, S. (2004). A statistical portrait of well-being in early adulthood. *Cross Currents: Child Trends Databank*, Issue 2, Publication #2004–18.

Bureau of Justice Statistics. (2006, September). *National crime victimization survey: Criminal victimization, 2005* (US Bureau of Justice Statistics Bulletin NCJ 214644). Washington, DC: US Department of Justice.

Bureau of Justice Statistics. (2007, August). *Black victims of violent crime* (Bureau of Justice Statistics Special Report NCJ 214258). Washington, DC: US Department of Justice.

Burton, L. M., Obedalliah, D. O., & Allison, K. (1996). Ethnographic insights on social context and adolescent development among inner-city African-American teens. In R. Jessor, A. Colby, & R. Shweder (Eds.), *Ethnography and human development: Context and meaning in social inquiry* (pp. 395–419). Chicago: University of Chicago Press.

Cauce, A. M., Coronado, N., & Watson, J. (1998). Conceptual, methodological, and statistical issues is culturally competent research. In M. Hernandez & R. Isaacs (Eds.), *Promoting cultural competence in children's mental health services*. Baltimore: Brookes.

Cauce, A. M., Hiraga, Y., Graves, D., Gonzales, N., Ryan-Finn, K., & Grove, K. (1996). African American mothers and their adolescent daughters: Closeness, conflict, and control. In B. J. Leadbeater & N. Way (Eds.), *Urban girls: Resisting stereotypes, creating identities* (pp. 100–116). New York: New York University Press.

Ceballo, R., & McLoyd, V. C. (2002). Social support and parenting in poor, dangerous neighborhoods. *Child Development, 73*, 1310–1321.

Center for Disease Control. (2007). Youth risk behavior surveillance—United States. *Morbidity & Mortality Weekly Report, 57*(SS-4), 1–131.

Charlton, B. (2007, February 5). Obama had multiethnic existence in Hawaii. *San Francisco Chronicle*.

Conger, R. D., Conger, K. J., Elder, G. H., Jr., Lorenz, F. O., & Simons, R. L. (1994). Economic stress, coercive family process and developmental problems of adolescents. *Child Development, 65*, 541–561.

Conger, K. J., Rueter, M. A., & Conger, R. D. (2000). The role of economic pressure in the lives of parents and their adolescents: The family stress model. In L. J. Crockett & R. J. Silbereisen (Eds.), *Negotiating adolescence in times of social change* (pp. 201–233). Cambridge: Cambridge University Press.

Conger, R. D., Ge, N., Elder, G. H., Lorenz, F. O., & Simons, R. L. (1994). Economic stress, coercive family process, and developmental problems of adolescents. *Child Development 65*, 541–561

Crane, J. (1991). The epidemic theory of ghettos and neighborhood effect on dropping out and teenage childbearing. *American Journal of Sociology, 96*, 1226–1259.

Dahl, R. (2004). Adolescent brain development: A period of vulnerabilities and opportunities. *Annals of the New York Academy of Sciences, 1021*, 1–22.

Deater-Deckard, K., Dodge, K. A., Bates, J. E., & Pettit, G. S. (1996). Physical discipline among African-American and European-American mothers: Links to children's externalizing behaviors. *Developmental Psychology, 32*, 1065–1072.

Dixon, S. V., Graber, J. A., & Brooks-Gunn, J. (2008). The roles of respect for parental authority and parenting practices in parent-child conflict among African American, Latino, and European American families. *Journal of Family Psychology, 22*, 1–11.

Duncan, G., & Raudenbush, S. W. (2002). Neighborhoods and adolescent development: How can we determine the links? In A. Booth & N. Crouter (Eds.), *Does it take a village? Community effects on children adolescents, and families*. State College, PA: Pennsylvania State University Press.

Editors, New York Times. (2009, July 22). The gates case and racial profiling. *New York Times*.

Feldman, S. S., & Eliott, G. R. (1990). *At the threshold: The developing adolescent*. Cambridge, MA: Harvard University Press.

Finkelhor, D., & Ormrod, R. (2000). *Characteristics of crimes against juveniles* (OJJDP Bulletin NCJ 179034). Washington, DC: Department of Justice, Office of Juvenile Justice and Delinquency Prevention.

Fox, H. B., McManus, M. A., Zarit, G. F., Cassedy, A. E., Bethell, C. D., & Read, D. (2007). *Racial and ethnic disparities in adolescent health and access to care*. Washington, DC: The National Alliance to Advance Adolescent Health Fact Sheet One.

Gandara, P. (1995). *Over the ivy walls: The educational mobility of low-income Chicanos*. Albany: SUNY Press.

Garbarino, J. (2001). An ecological perspective on the effects of violence on children. *Journal of Community Psychology, 29*, 361–378.

Garcia Coll, C., Lamberty, G., Jenkins, R., McAdoo, H. P., Crnic, K., Wasik, B. H., et al. (1996). An integrative model for the study of developmental competencies in minority children. *Child Development, 5*, 1891–1914.

Gibson, C. L., Morris, S. Z., & Beaver, K. M. (2009). Secondary exposure to violence during childhood and adolescence: Does neighborhood context matter? *Justice Quarterly, 26*, 30–57.

Gonzales, N., Cauce, A. M., & Mason, C. (1996). Interobserver agreement in the assessment of parental behavior and parent-adolescent conflict: African American mothers, daughters, and independent observers. *Child Development, 67*, 1483–1498.

Gonzalez, R., & Padilla, A. M. (1997). The academic resilience of Mexican American high school students. *Hispanic Journal of Behavioral Sciences, 19*, 301–317.

Gordon-Larsen, P., Nelson, M. C., Page, P., & Popkin, B. M. (2006). Inequality in the build environment underlies key health disparities in physical activity and obesity. *Pediatrics, 117*, 417–424.

Haynie, D. L., Silver, E., & Teasdale, B. (2006). Neighborhood characteristics, peer networks, and adolescent violence. *Journal of Quantitative Criminology, 22*, 147–169.

Hernandez, D. J. (1993). *America's children: Resources from family, government, and the economy*. New York: Russell Sage Foundation.

Hovey, J. D., & King, C. A. (1996). Acculturative stress, depression, and suicidal ideation among immigrant and second generation Latino adolescents. *Journal of the American Academy of Child and Adolescent Psychiatry, 35*, 1183–1192.

Huston, A., Duncan, G., Granger, R., Bos, H., McLoyd, V. C., Mistry, R., et al. (2001). Work-based anti-poverty programs for parents can enhance the school performance and social behavior of children. *Child Development, 72*, 318–336.

Israel, B. A., Schulz, A. J., Estrada-Martinez, L., Zenk, S. N., Viruell-Fuentes, E., Villarruel, A. M., et al. (2006). Engaging community residents in assessing urban environments and their implications for health. *Journal of Urban Health, 83*, 523–539.

Jargowsky, P. A. (1997). *Poverty and place: Ghettos, barrios, and the American city.* New York: Russell Sage Foundation.

Jargowsky, P. A., & Bane, M. J. (1991). Ghetto poverty in the United States, 1970–1980. In C. Jencks & P. E. Peterson (Eds.), *The urban underclass* (pp. 235–273). Washington, DC: The Brookings Institution.

Jarrett, R. L. (1997). African American family and parenting strategies in impoverished neighborhoods. *Qualitative Sociology, 20*, 275–288.

Jarrett, R. L. (1999). Successful parenting in high-risk neighborhoods. *The Future of Children: When School is Out, 9*, 45–50.

Katz, S. R. (1999). Teaching in tensions: Immigrant youth, their teachers, and the structures of schooling. *Teachers College Record, 4*, 809–840.

Kessler, R. C., Avenevoli, S., Costello, E. J., Green, J. G., Gruber, M. J., Heeringa, S., et al. (2009). Design and field procedures in the US National Comorbidity Survey Replication adolescent supplement (NCS-A). *International Journal of Methods in Psychiatric Research, 18*, 69–83.

Kessler, R. C., & Merkikangas, K. R. (2004). The National Comorbidity Survey Replication (NCS-R): Background and aims. *International Journal of Methods in Psychiatric Research, 13*, 60–69.

Loeber, R., & Farrington, D. P. (2001). *Child delinquents: Developmental intervention and service needs.* Thousand Oaks, CA: Sage.

Loeber, R., & Stouthamer-Loeber, M. (1996). The development of offending. *Criminal Justice and Behavior, 23*, 12–24.

Loukas, A., Prelow, H. M., Suizzo, M. A., & Allua, S. (2008). Mothering and peer associations mediate cumulative risk effects for Latino youth. *Journal of Marriage and Family, 70*, 76–85.

Luthar, S. S. (1999). Poverty and children's adjustment. Newbury Park, CA: Sage.

Luthar, S. S., Cicchetti, D., & Becker, B. (2000). The construct of resilience: A critical evaluation and guidelines for future work. *Child Development, 71*, 543–562.

Martin, J. A., Hamilton, B. E., Sutton, P. D., Ventura, S. J., Menacker, F. J., Kirmeyer, S., et al. (2009). *Births: Final data for 2006* (National Vital Statistics Reports, 57). Hyattsville, MD: National Center for Health Statistics.

Mason, C. A., Cauce, A. M., & Gonzales, N. (1997). Parents and peers in the lives of African-American adolescents: An interactive approach to the study of problem behavior. In R. W. Taylor & M. C. Wang (Eds.), *Social and emotional adjustment and family relations in ethnic minority families.* Mahwah, NJ: Lawrence Erlbaum Associates.

Mason, C. A., Cauce, A. M., Gonzales, N., & Hiraga, Y. (1994). Adolescent problem behavior: The effect of peers and the moderating role of father absence and the mother-child relationship. *American Journal of Community Psychology, 22*, 723–743.

Mason, C. A., Cauce, A. M., Gonzales, N., & Hiraga, Y. (1996). Neither too sweet nor too sour: Problem peers, maternal control, and problem behavior in African American adolescents. *Child Development, 67*, 2115–2130.

Mason, C. A., Walker-Barnes, C. J., Tu, S., Simons, J., & Martinez-Arrue, R. (2004). Ethnic differences in the affective meaning of parental control behaviors. *Journal of Primary Prevention, 25*, 59–79.

Masten, A. S., & Obradović, J. (2006). Competence and resilience in development. *Annals of the New York Academy of Sciences, 1094*, 13–27.

McLoyd, V. C. (1998). Socioeconomic disadvantage and child development. *American Psychologist, 53*, 185–204.

McLoyd, V. C., Cauce, A. M., Takeuchi, D., & Wilson, L. (2000). Marital processes and parental socialization in families of color: A decade review of research. *Journal of Marriage and the Family, 62*, 1070–1093.

McLoyd, V. C., & Smith, J. (2002). Physical discipline and behavior problems in African American, European American, and Latino children: Emotional support as a moderator. *Journal of Marriage and the Family, 64*, 40–53.

Mengesha, L. (2009). *The only black student*. Seattle, WA: Mengesha Publishing.

Meyers, S. A., Miller, C. (2004). Direct, mediated, moderated, and cumulative relations between neighborhood characteristics and adolescent outcomes. *Adolescence, 39*, 935–951.

Mistry, R., Vandewater, E., Huston, A., & McLoyd, V. C. (2002). Economic well-being and children's social adjustment: The role of family process in an ethnically diverse low-income sample. *Child Development, 73*, 935–951.

Morland, K., Wing, S., Roux, A. D., & Poole, C. (2002). Neighborhood characteristics associated with the location of food store and food service places. *American Journal of Preventive Medicine, 22*, 23–29.

National Center for Education Statistics. (2009, April). *Indicators of school crime and safety: 2008*. Washington, DC: US Department of Education, US Department of Justice Office of Justice Programs. NCES 2009-022, NCJ 226343.

Obama, B. (1995, 2004). *Dreams from my father: A story of race and inheritance*. New York: Three Rivers Press.

O'Donnell, D., Schwab-Stone, M., & Muyeed, A. (2002). Multidimensional resilience in urban children exposed to community violence. *Child Development, 73*, 1265–1282.

Office of Justice Programs. (2009, April). *Juvenile arrests 2007* (Juvenile Justice Bulletin). Washington, DC: U.S. Department of Justice.

Ogden, C. L., Carroll, M. D., Curtin, L. R., McDowell, M. A., Tabak, C. J., & Flegal, K. M. (2006). Prevalence of overweight and obesity in the United States, 1999–2004. *Journal of the American Medical Association, 295*, 1549–1555.

Parke, R. D. (2004). Fathers, families, and the future: A plethora of plausible predictions. *Merrill-Palmer Quarterly, 50*, 456–470.

Patthey-Chavez, G. G. (1993). High school as an arena for cultural conflict and acculturation for Latino Angelinos. *Anthropology and Education Quarterly, 24*, 33–60.

Perkins, C. A. (1997, September). *Age patterns of victims of serious crimes*. Washington, DC: Bureau of Justice Statistics, U.S. Department of Justice, NCJ-162031.

Pittman, L. D., & Chase-Lansdale, P. L. (2001). African American adolescent girls in impoverished communities: Parenting style and adolescent outcomes. *Journal of Research on Adolescence, 11*, 199–224.

Proctor, B. D., & Dalakar, J. (2002). *Poverty in the United States: 2001. Current population reports* (Series P60-219). Washington, DC: Department of Commerce, US Census Bureau.

Quane, J. M., & Rankin, B. H. (1998). Neighborhood poverty, family characteristics, and commitment to mainstream goals. *Journal of Family Issues, 19*, 769–794.

Rankin, B. H., & Quane, J. M. (2002). Social contexts and urban adolescent outcomes: The interrelated effects of neighborhoods, families, and peers on African American youth. *Social Problems, 49*, 79–100.

Roberts, S. (2008, August 7). Minorities often a majority of the population under 20. *New York Times*.

Roche, K. M., Ensmiger, M. E., & Cherlin, A. J. (2007). Variations in parenting and adolescent outcomes among African American and Latino families living in low-income, urban areas. *Journal of Family Issues, 28*, 882–909.

Roosa, M., Weaver, S. R., White, R. M. B., Tien, J., Knight, G. P., Gonzales, N., et al. (2009). Family and neighborhood fit or misfit and the adaptation of Mexican Americans. *American Journal of Community Psychology, 44*, 15–27.

Rueschenberg, E., & Buriel, R. (1989). Mexican American family functioning and acculturation: A family systems perspective. *Hispanic Journal of Behavioral Sciences, 11*, 232–244.

Sabogal, F., Marín, G., Otero-Sabogal, R., Marín, B. V., & Pérez-Stable, E. J. (1987). Hispanic familism and acculturation: What changes and what doesn't? *Hispanic Journal of Behavioral Sciences, 9*, 397–412.

Sampson, R. J., & Sharkey, P. (2008). Neighborhood selection and the social reproduction of concentrated racial inequality. *Demography, 45*, 1–29.

Sharkey, P. (2009). *Neighborhood and the black-white mobility gap.* Washington, DC: The Economic Mobility Project: An Initiative of the Pew Charitable Trusts.

Smith, C., & Thornberry., T. P. (1995). The relationship between childhood maltreatment and adolescent involvement in delinquency and drug use. *Criminology, 33*, 451–481.

Takeuchi, D., Alegria, M., Jackson, J. S., & Williams, D. R. (2007). Immigration and mental health: Diverse findings in Asian, Black, and Latino populations. *American Journal of Public Health, 97*, 11–12.

Thornberry, T. P., & Krohn, M. D. (2003). *Taking stock of delinquency: An overview of findings from contemporary longitudinal studies.* New York: Kluwe Academic/Plenum Press.

Timberlake, J. M. (2006). *Racial and ethnic inequality in the duration of children's exposure to neighborhood poverty and affluence* (Working Paper available at http://www.npc.umich.edu/publications/working_papers/index.php?low_date=2006-01-01&high_date=2006-12-31).

Timberlake, J., & Michael, J. (2006, August 10). *Children's exposure to neighbourhood poverty and affluence in the United States, 1990–2000.* Paper presented at the annual meeting of the American Sociological Association, Montreal Convention Center, Montreal, QC, Canada.

United States Department of Labor. (1965, March). *The Negro family: The case for national action (The Moynihan Report).* Washington, DC: Author.

Villarruel, A. (1998). Cultural influences on the sexual attitudes, beliefs, and norms of young Latina adolescents. *Journal of the Society of Pediatric Nurses, 3*, 69–79.

Wen, M., Browning, C. R., & Cagney, K. A. (2003). Poverty, affluence, and income inequality: Neighborhood economic structure and its implications for health. *Social Science and Medicine, 57*, 843–860.

Wirt, J., Choy, S., Rooney, P., Provasnik, S., Sen, A., & Tobin, R. (2006). *The condition of education 2006* (NCES 2006-071). U.S. Department of Education, National Center for Education Statistics. Washington, DC: US Government Printing Office, table 21–1.

How Money Matters for Children's Socioemotional Adjustment: Family Processes and Parental Investment

Vonnie C. McLoyd

Numerous studies conducted by researchers in public health, psychology, and sociology have found that children and adolescents from disadvantaged families (e.g., "officially poor" families, families with low income-to-needs ratios) are at an increased risk of mental health problems, including depressive symptomatology, hostility, difficulties in peer relations, low self-esteem, and drug use (Bolger, Patterson, & Thompson, 1995; Brooks-Gunn & Furstenberg, 1989; Currie & Lin, 2007; Elder, Nguyen, & Caspi, 1985; Goodman, 1999; Goosby, 2007; Strohschein, 2005; Wadsworth, Raviv, Compas, & Connor-Smith, 2005).[1] These difficulties are intensified among children who experience longer spells of poverty (Bolger et al., 1995; Goosby, 2007). Direct associations between economic disadvantage and child mental health are most commonly found when mothers, teachers, clinicians, and peers are informants about the child's adjustment. However, when children report on their own mental health, often only indirect associations, mediated through the actions of parents, are found (e.g., Conger, Ge, Elder, Lorenz, & Simons, 1994; McLoyd, Jayaratne, Ceballo, & Borquez, 1994).

Stressors and the reactions they evoke are central constructs in numerous models that scholars have articulated to explain the relationship between family-level economic disadvantage and child mental health. They include the family stress model (Conger et al., 1992; Elder, 1974), stress-vulnerability response models (e.g., Sinha, 2001), bioecological models (Bronfenbrenner & Ceci, 1994), and cumulative stress models emphasizing allostatic load, a physiologic marker of cumulative wear and tear on the body caused by repeated mobilization of multiple physiological response

V.C. McLoyd (✉)
Department of Psychology, University of North Carolina, Chapel Hill, NC 27599, USA
e-mail: vcmcloyd@unc.edu

Paper prepared for an edited volume based on a presentation at the 57th Annual Nebraska Symposium on Motivation: *Motivation and Health: Addressing Youth Health Disparities in the Twenty First Century*, University of Nebraska, Lincoln, April 16, 2009, organized by Gustavo Carlo, Lisa Crockett, and Miguel Carranza.

[1] For convenience, the term "children" is used to refer to children and adolescents. When the distinction between these two developmental periods is critical, the applicable term is used.

systems (Evans, Kim, Ting, Tesher, & Shannas, 2007; for a brief discussion of these models, see McLoyd et al., 2009).

Because of the myriad stressors attendant to poverty and low-income status, the explanatory emphasis on stressors is not surprising. Neither poverty nor low-income is a unitary variable or distinct event. Rather, they are a conglomerate of stressful conditions and events, many of which are outside personal control, especially if poverty or low-income status is chronic. Individuals who are poor or near-poor often are confronted with an unremitting succession of negative life events (e.g., eviction, physical illness, criminal assault) in the context of a daunting array of adverse life conditions (e.g., inadequate housing, dangerous neighborhoods, proximity to toxic waste dumps, elevated levels of exposure to lead, pesticides, ambient air pollution, radon) that together increase the exigencies of day-to-day existence (Evans, 2004). Because of limited financial resources, negative life events often precipitate additional crises. Problems in one domain can exacerbate or create problems in another domain. Because of this high contagion of stressors, chronic economic disadvantage is most appropriately viewed as a pervasive, rather than bounded, stressor that restricts choices in virtually all domains of life (e.g., choice of neighborhood, school, educational and recreational activities; Makosky, 1982; McLoyd, 1990).

This chapter focuses attention on the family stress model, one of the most widely examined explanations for the association between economic disadvantage and child mental health. Following a brief discussion of this model and corroborating evidence from correlational research, I summarize research that my colleagues and I have conducted that extends aspects of the family stress model. I then focus attention on the New Hope program, an antipoverty, work-based intervention that raised family income above the poverty threshold through earnings supplements and thereby offered an opportunity to assess the robustness of the family stress model within an experimental, random assignment design. To put the effects of New Hope in broader perspective, the findings of two syntheses of the effects of an array of employment-based welfare and antipoverty experiments are reviewed. Of special interest is whether findings from experiments that provided earnings supplements such as New Hope converge with those from correlational studies linking family income to child mental health through family processes. The chapter concludes with a discussion of directions for future research.

Linking Economic Disadvantage and Child Mental Health: The Family Stress Model

The core assumption of the family stress model is that economic hardship adversely affects children's psychological adjustment indirectly through its impact on the parent's behavior toward the child. It is posited that economic stress produces feelings of economic strain that impair parents' mental health, which in turn, undermines the quality of parenting (e.g., higher levels of punitive and inconsistent discipline, lower levels of parental nurturance, monitoring, supervision, and support of the child). The model derives from Elder's seminal studies of the effects on European-American families of parental job and income loss during the Great Depression (Elder, 1974; Elder et al., 1985). In these studies, Elder and his colleagues found few direct effects of economic hardship on children's behavior and psychological functioning. Rather, the adverse effects of economic hardship were produced indirectly, through negative effects on fathers' psychological functioning and parenting behaviors. Fathers who sustained heavy financial loss became more irritable, tense, and explosive, which increased their tendency to be punitive, rejecting, and inconsistent in disciplining their children. In turn, these negative fathering behaviors were predictive of emotional difficulties in children.

Studies of contemporary families have generated robust support for this model. These studies document associations between economic stress and psychological distress in parents (e.g., more depressive symptoms, lower sense of mastery). Moreover, they demonstrate that parental psychological distress and family processes such as spousal relations, parenting behaviors, and parent-child relations mediate the relation between economic hardship and psychosocial outcomes such as internalizing and externalizing behavior in children and adolescents and that these relations generally hold across ethnicity, socioeconomic background, and geographic context (i.e., rural, urban) (e.g., Bolger et al., 1995; Brody et al., 1994; Conger et al., 1992, 1994, 2002; Goosby, 2007; McLoyd et al., 1994; Mistry, Vandewater, Huston, & McLoyd, 2002; Taylor, Rodriguez, Seaton, & Dominguez, 2004).

Elaborations of the Family Stress Model

In addition to examining parenting behavior as a mediator of the link between economic stress and children's mental health (Conger et al., 2002; McLoyd et al., 1994; Mistry et al., 2002), my colleagues and I have focused attention on linkages among neighborhood factors, parents' psychological functioning, and parenting behavior to understand better parenting behavior and children's development in relation to ecological niches. In particular, we have examined neighborhood factors as mediators and moderators of particular linkages in the family stress model. We have concentrated on African American families living in urban communities because of the comparatively high prevalence of economic stress among these families and because they are an understudied segment of the population with respect to the family stress model. Of the studies testing the family stress model in African American families, most focus on samples drawn from rural and suburban areas (Brody & Flor, 1998; Brody et al., 1994, 1995; Conger et al., 2002; Gutman & Eccles, 1999). Only a handful are based on African American families living in urban areas (e.g., Jackson, Brooks-Gunn, Huang, & Glassman, 2000; McLoyd et al., 1994; Taylor et al., 2004).

Wilson's (1987) analysis of historical changes in the spatial concentration of poverty in inner-city African American neighborhoods wrought by structural changes in the economy generated keen interest in the demographics and consequences of the context of childhood poverty. He pondered whether poor children's development is conditioned by variation in the prevalence of economic hardship in their respective neighborhoods (e.g., percentage of poverty, unemployment, welfare receipt). During the 1970s and 1980s, poor African American children were far more likely than poor non-Hispanic white children to live in high-poverty neighborhoods (i.e., neighborhoods in which at least 40% of the residents were poor) where jobs, high-quality public and private services (e.g., child care, schools, parks, community centers, youth organizations), and informal social supports are less accessible (Duncan, 1991; Shinn & Gillespie, 1994; Wilson, 1987). This pattern has persisted, although the disparities appear to have narrowed since that time. The 1990s brought declines in the concentration of poverty. The share of the metropolitan poor who lived in high-poverty census tracts dropped from 17% in 1980s to 12% in 2000. This period was also marked by changes in the composition of concentrated poverty by race. In particular, the share of all high-poverty tracts with predominantly (more than 60%) African American populations declined from 48% in 1980 to 39% in 2000, with compensating increases occurring in the shares that were predominantly Hispanic (Kingsley & Pettit, 2003). In 2000, about 54% of African American children who were officially poor lived in high-poverty neighborhoods (as assessed in 1989), compared to 51% of poor Hispanic children and 47% of poor non-Hispanic White children (U.S. Department of Health & Human Services, 2002).

Efforts to understand the mental health consequences of living in economically depressed urban neighborhoods have concentrated on three types of neighborhood characteristics in relation to mental health outcomes: structural characteristics (e.g., SES, racial/ethnic composition, residential patterns) social (e.g., drug trade, corner gangs, public drunkenness) and physical (e.g., abandoned buildings, vandalism, litter) incivilities, and elements of the ambient and built environment (e.g., noise, crowding, pollution, high-rise buildings). Correlational studies have documented positive relations between (a) neighborhood-level social/physical incivilities and fear of criminal victimization (construed by some researchers as a mental health outcome), and (b) perception of crime and poor mental health (e.g., depressive symptoms, anxiety, and somatization) (see Wandersman & Nation for a discussion of this research).

Moreover, experimental research suggests causal links between neighborhood conditions and parental mental health. Moving to Opportunity (MTO) program is a randomized housing mobility experiment conducted by the U.S. Department of Housing and Urban Development that helps poor urban families (about 2/3 are African American; over 90% are single-parent families) move out of poor, inner-city high-risk neighborhoods and settle in low-poverty neighborhoods (where less than 10% of the population is poor). A recent interim evaluation of the experiment at the 3-year follow-up found that the experimental group (i.e., those given housing vouchers enabling them to move to private housing in low-poverty neighborhoods), compared to the control group (those who did not receive vouchers and remained in public housing), reported less physical and social disorder in their neighborhoods (e.g., presence of trash, graffiti, abandoned buildings, loitering, and public drinking/drug use or dealing), reductions in the likelihood of observing or being victims of crime, increases in their perception of safety in and around their homes, greater satisfaction with their neighborhoods (corroborated by interviewers' ratings of families' immediate external environment), and fewer depressive and distress symptoms (Leventhal & Brooks-Gunn, 2003; Orr et al., 2003). Mental health also improved among daughters (reductions in psychological distress, generalized anxiety, and risky behaviors such as marijuana use, smoking), but not sons.

(a) Neighborhood stress as a mediator of the income-psychological distress link. In a study of 305 African American families living in inner city neighborhoods, 40% of whom had incomes at or below the U.S. poverty threshold, we tested an expanded version of the family stress model that hypothesized both financial strain and neighborhood stress as mediators of the link between low-income and parental psychological distress (Gutman, McLoyd, & Toyokawa, 2005). Financial strain (e.g., worrying about not having money) is a construct that gives psychological meaning to objective indicators of economic difficulty or insufficient income relative to needs, whereas neighborhood stress is a construct that captures respondents' perception of disorder and neglect in their neighborhood. Our measure of neighborhood stress assessed perceptions of neighborhood problems (e.g., high unemployment, vandalism, and drug use or drug dealing in the open), barriers to social services (e.g., perceived unavailability in the neighborhood of decent health and social services for children), low social control (e.g., the perception that it is unlikely that a neighbor would intervene or call police if someone was breaking into the respondent's home in plain sight), and chances of success for adolescents residing in the neighborhood (e.g., graduating from high school; completing college; finding a stable, well-paying job as an adult; entering the military).

As predicted, parents' (90% were mothers) perceptions of neighborhood-level problems mediated the link between family income and parental psychological distress independently of perceived financial strain. Parents with lower income-to-need ratios reported more neighborhood stress, independently of financial strain, and both neighborhood stress and financial strain predicted higher levels of psychological distress in parents (i.e., anxiety, depression, anger). Parents experiencing more psychological distress had more negative and less positive parent-adolescent relations, which in turn, predicted higher negative and less positive adjustment in adolescents.

The findings suggest that efforts to strengthen parenting behavior and improve parent and adolescent adjustment may be bolstered by practices and policies that reduce neighborhood stress. Interventions based on organizational development principles have been found to improve the efficacy (e.g., to reduce vandalism and public drunkenness, increase neighboring and a sense of community) and viability of block organizations, but evaluations of these interventions have not assessed impacts on individual-level psychological functioning (Wandersman & Nation, 1998). We know from the MTO experiment, discussed previously, that improvements in neighborhood conditions benefit parents' mental health (e.g., Leventhal & Brooks-Gunn, 2003). Given evidence linking parents' mental health and parenting behavior (McLoyd, 1990), it is plausible that improvements in neighborhood conditions will also promote positive parenting or lessen negative parenting.

(b) Neighborhood disadvantage as a moderator of the psychological distress-parenting link. In a second study, we focused on ineffective child management as a correlate of maternal psychological distress and assessed whether neighborhood disadvantage—defined in terms of perceived social control, safety, and disorganization—moderated the strength of this association (McLoyd, Kaplan, & Hardaway, 2010). In addition to exhibiting diminished involvement, nurturance, and sensitivity and more punitive behaviors toward their children, mothers experiencing higher levels of psychological distress also perceive their disciplinary strategies to be less effective and are less consistent in following through on their requests when the child does not comply (Conger, Patterson, & Ge, 1995; Zelkowitz, 1982). Because there is strong evidence that inconsistent-harsh parenting and ineffective discipline (e.g., child getting away with things the parent thinks should have been punished; use of punishment strategies that have no deterrent effect) contribute to rule-breaking behavior and conduct disorder in children (e.g., Capaldi, Pears, Patterson, & Owen, 2003; Kim et al., 2003; Stanger, Dumenci, Kamon, & Burstein, 2004), understanding the processes that shape these parenting behaviors is important.

Living in neighborhoods where threats to personal safety are salient, where one is less able to count on neighbors to foil crimes and thwart acts that threaten personal safety, and where abandoned, boarded up houses or buildings, graffiti, and garbage on streets and sidewalks are commonplace arguably constitutes a pervasive, chronic stressor. As such, it is likely to not only increase feelings of psychological distress, but also increase the likelihood that psychological distress will adversely affect child management, in effect, amplifying the relation between psychological distress and child management. We found evidence for this moderating effect in a longitudinal study of over 500 low-income families followed over a period of 8 years. Mothers experiencing more psychological distress reported higher levels of ineffective child management, even controlling for the effects of ineffective child management and child behavior problems in previous years. Moreover, maternal psychological distress was significantly and positively related to ineffective child management only among those living in neighborhoods with low levels of social control. In high social control neighborhoods, maternal psychological distress was unrelated to ineffective child management.

Conceptualizing psychological distress as a risk factor for inept child management, our findings are consistent with other research suggesting that the adverse effects of risk factors are amplified in more pernicious, resource-poor contexts and diminished in more benign contexts (Dubow, Edwards, & Ippolito, 1997; Lynam et al., 2000; Rankin & Quane, 2002). They are also consistent with recent evidence that variation in the context where low-income families live influences the degree of association between maternal psychological functioning and parenting. For example, in their study of African American single mothers, Kotchick, Dorsey, and Heller (2005) found that neighborhood stress adversely affected parenting through increases in psychological distress to a greater extent among mothers who perceived lower social support in their communities than among mothers who perceived higher social support.

(c) Neighborhood disadvantage as a moderator of the link between social support and parenting. In a third study, we investigated whether neighborhood disadvantage influences the relation between mothers' social support and parenting behavior in a sample of poor, single African American mothers and their adolescent children residing in an economically depressed Midwestern city. Our measure of neighborhood disadvantage was based on interview data from mothers and children, as well as objective data about respondents' neighborhoods (e.g., crime statistics) (Ceballo & McLoyd, 2002). There is considerable evidence that greater access to social support is associated with more nurturant and less punitive parenting strategies (McLoyd, 1990). At the most extreme end of the continuum, isolation from social networks and support is repeatedly associated with child abuse and neglect among poor families (Garbarino, 1977; Garbarino & Sherman, 1980; Wandersman & Nation). In contrast, several studies have found that support systems serve as protective moderators of negative life stressors, enhancing adults' psychological well-being and parenting (Campbell & Lee, 1992; Dressler, 1985; Taylor, Casten, & Flickinger, 1993). Mothers with higher levels of social support are generally more sensitive, nurturant, and consistent in their parenting and less likely to use punitive strategies such as scolding and ridiculing. Emotional and practical support may enhance maternal behavior by protecting against depression and fostering positive parent-child relations (McLoyd, 1990, 1998).

In our study, neighborhood disadvantage was based on three indicators: (a) maternal ratings of neighborhood quality in terms of police protection, quality of neighborhood schools, public transportation, crime, drug activity, and community involvement, (b) violent crime rates based on statistics provided by the city's police department on the number of selected crimes (murder, rape, robbery, assault, breaking and entering, larceny, auto theft, arson) committed in the respondents' reporting area (respondents lived in 30 of the 64 police-reporting area in the city), and (c) percentage of families living in poverty in the respondent's census tract (respondents resided in 20 of the 40 census tracts in the city). We found that neighborhood conditions moderated the relation between social support and parenting behaviors. As neighborhood conditions worsened (e.g., lower ratings of neighborhood by respondents, higher crime rates), the *positive* relation between emotional support and mothers' nurturant parenting decreased. In parallel fashion, as the surrounding environments became poorer and more dangerous, the strength of the *negative* relation between instrumental support and reliance on punishment decreased as well. In short, the beneficial effects of social support on parenting, often conceptualized as a protective factor, were diminished in more disadvantaged neighborhoods (Ceballo & McLoyd, 2002).

If we conceive of living in a high-risk neighborhood as a chronic stressor, our findings appear consistent with evidence that social support is less effective in buffering the distress associated with chronic economic hardship, as compared to the distress of isolated negative life events, among young African American women (Dressler, 1985). The positive effects of social support may be reduced in high-risk neighborhoods partly because the social networks of mothers in disadvantaged neighborhoods are often comprised of individuals who themselves are experiencing high levels of psychological distress due to numerous negative life events and conditions. Their needs and demands may negate the support that they provide. Additionally, the psychological and physical threats that high-risk neighborhoods pose may simply overwhelm whatever positive benefits social support has on parenting in more benign contexts. Almost three decades earlier, Belle (1982) cautioned that the ameliorative qualities of social support may be reduced in high-risk neighborhoods. Her qualitative study of single, low-income African American mothers residing in impoverished neighborhoods suggested that receipt of social support is not a uniformly positive process because providers of support often are themselves sources of stress. A majority of mothers in her study described relations with friends and extended family as such, and especially prized their solitary independence as a result.

Summarizing, our tests of extensions of the family stress model indicate that (a) neighborhood-level problems mediate the link between family income and parental psychological distress independently of perceived financial strain, (b) the relation between maternal psychological distress and inept child management is amplified in neighborhoods where social control is low, and (c) the beneficial effects of social support on parenting are diminished in more disadvantaged neighborhood.

Tests of the family stress model discussed thus far have relied on correlational data. A recent generation of experimental studies assessing the effects of different welfare and employment policies on child well-being offered opportunities to test the robustness of this model within an experimental, random assignment design. The next section summarizes the findings from an exemplar of these experimental studies—the New Hope Project.

The New Hope Project: Assessing the Family Stress Model in an Antipoverty Experiment

Critics of Aid to Families with Dependent Children (AFDC) have long argued that the program mires families in poverty because it encourages out-of-wedlock births and contains strong disincentives to work, yet does not provide benefits sufficient to lift families out of poverty (Blank & Blum, 1997; Duncan, Huston, & Weisner, 2007). By the early 1990s, this argument had gained widespread acceptance among policymakers, and political resolve to curtail public welfare reached unprecedented levels (Morris, Huston, Duncan, Crosby, & Bos, 2001). A critical outcome of this resolve was passage of The Personal Responsibility and Work Opportunity Reconciliation Act (PRWORA) in 1996. This law ended entitlement to cash assistance for poor families, established a non-entitlement program (Temporary Assistance to Needy Families—TANF), set time limits on eligibility for assistance, and created strong work requirements for families that received temporary assistance (Greenberg et al., 2002).

Several years prior to passage of this law, a large number of states had received waivers of AFDC rules to experiment with changes in welfare provisions. States' receipt of waivers from the federal government was conditional on use of a random assignment design and evaluation of proposed programs (Morris et al., 2001). Because the avowed purpose of most welfare policies is promotion of child well-being, many of these evaluations examined effects on children. States mixed and matched several kinds of welfare and employment policies, including policies intended to promote employment through penalties and incentives. The resulting diversity of programs provided an opportunity to assess the comparative effects of different program features on child well-being and development. Because these experimental programs anticipated key elements of PRWORA, they offered lessons about the potential effects on children of welfare reform policies legislated after PRWORA (Morris et al., 2001). One of these pre-PRWORA programs was New Hope, an anti-poverty, work-based program established in 1994 in inner-city Milwaukee. Below, I discuss the components of this program, our hypothesized model of how it would impact families and children, and the effects of the program at three time-points.

Goals and Components of New Hope

New Hope's goal was to improve the lives of low-income families by increasing employment and income. Operated by a community-based nonprofit organization and funded by a consortium of local, state, and national organizations, the state of Wisconsin, and the federal government, New Hope functioned outside the existing public welfare assistance system, but was designed to be replicable as government policy. Four main principles guided the program: (a) people who are willing to work full-time should have the opportunity to do so; (b) people who work full-time should not be poor; (c) people should have an incentive to increase earnings; and (d) regular employment should be financially more rewarding than subsidized employment or other forms of public assistance (Bos et al., 1999).

In order to participate in the New Hope program, adults had to be living in one of two zip-code defined neighborhoods in Milwaukee's poorest areas, be at least 18 years old, be willing and able to work at least 30 hr/week and have a household income that was at or below 150% of the federally defined poverty level. When participants initially applied to the program, over 50% were unemployed and approximately 80% were receiving benefits in the form of AFDC, food stamps, Medicaid or other general assistance. Most of the participants were single mothers who had never married. Approximately 10% were married and living with their spouse. Applicants were randomly assigned to either the program group or control group through a lottery process. Both groups were eligible for federal and state public assistance, but only the program group members had access to the additional New Hope benefits (Bos et al., 1999).

Each New Hope participant was eligible for benefits for a total of 3 years, from 1994 to 1997. Benefits were reflective of the program's guiding principles. First, participants were provided individualized job search assistance. Those unable to find employment in the regular job market after 8 weeks were provided a community service job in a nonprofit organization. Participants who were employed but were not working 30 hr/week were also eligible for community service jobs. In addition to employment benefits, participants in the New Hope program who met the minimum 30 hr/work requirement were given earnings supplements if their household income was still below 200% of the poverty line. Participants also qualified for both the federal and Wisconsin Earned Tax Income Credits (EITC). These benefits ensured that the participants' household income was at or above the federal poverty line. Benefits also included health care subsidies for participants who did not receive health insurance coverage from their employer or through Medicaid.

Participants with children aged 13 or younger were provided financial assistance to help cover the cost of child care. In order to receive the monetary support, participants had to enroll their children in child care homes or centers that were either state-licensed or county certified. Finally, New Hope offered informational, instrumental, and emotional support to participants. Each participant was assigned a staff representative who provided information about New Hope benefits and related issues. Staff were trained to be respectful and supportive in all of their interactions with project participations.

Although New Hope was conceived as an alternative to the existing public welfare system, many participants in the program group continued to use public assistance or Medicaid in addition to or instead of New Hope benefits. For example, 2 years after entering the program, 24% of New Hope families in the Child and Family sample (described below) received AFDC, 46% received food stamps, and 29% received Special Supplemental Nutrition Program for Women, Infants and Children [WIC] benefits. Consequently, the evaluation of New Hope provides insight into what would happen if we added the supports available in New Hope *on top of existing policies and programs*, not what would happen if the existing welfare system was *replaced* with a work-based set of supports like those that New Hope provided (Bos et al., 1999).

The total sample of participants consisted of 1,357 adults (679 program group members; 678 control group members). The findings reported in this chapter pertain to a subsample of the full sample. This subsample, the focus of the New Hope "Child and Family Study," consisted of all participants who had at least one child between the ages of 1 and 10 years old (379 program group members; 366 control group members). If a family had multiple children in the age range, two focal children were chosen randomly to participate in the surveys, with the exception that preference was given to opposite-sex siblings. There were a total of 913 focal children (447 were in the program group).

Hypothesized Pathways of Influence

The conceptual model guiding the New Hope evaluation, presented in Fig. 1, was based on existing research. New Hope was expected to positively affect children's socioemotional adjustment and educational achievement through multiple pathways, namely increases in family income and parental employment, and positive

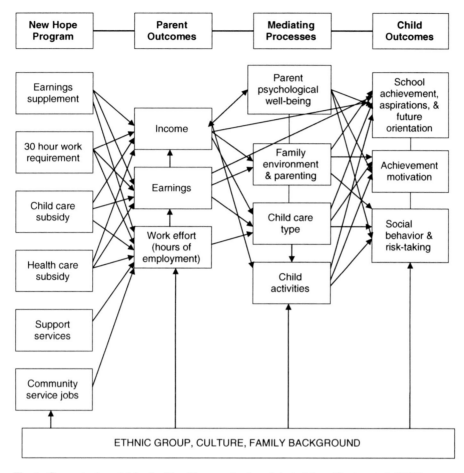

Fig. 1 Conceptual model for the New Hope evaluation. Adapted from Huston et al. (2003)

changes in parenting behaviors, child care settings and children's participation in organized, adult supervised activities. Each of these pathways is briefly discussed below.

Income and employment. An abundance of studies have linked higher family income to numerous indicators of adaptive functioning in children, including positive social behavior, psychological well-being, and academic achievement (Duncan & Brooks-Gunn, 1997; Hill & Sandford, 1995; Huston, 1991; Korenman, Miller, & Sjaastad, 1995). Additionally, in random assignment experiments conducted in the 1960s and 1970s that provided experimental families with a minimum level of income, elementary school children in the program group showed improved academic achievement when compared to the control group at some of the sites (Institute for Research on Poverty, 1976; Kershaw & Fair, 1976; Salkind & Haskins, 1982).

How increases in maternal employment expected from New Hope might affect children was less clear. More hours of maternal employment might reduce the amount of time that children have with their mother, but also provide positive benefits such as improved economic well-being, less financial stress, and a model of achievement for the child. Findings from studies of the effects of maternal employment on children in low-income families are mixed. Some studies have found no impacts on children (Cherry & Eaton, 1997; Desai, Chase-Lansdale, & Michael, 1989), while others have found that maternal employment is positively associated with children's social adjustment and academic achievement (e.g., Milne, Myers, Rosenthal, & Ginsburg, 1986; Vandell & Ramanan, 1992). Negative effects are more likely if children are left alone or placed in inadequate child care; if mothers enter jobs with low complexity (i.e., routine, repetitive activities with little opportunity for initiative; Parcel & Menaghan, 1997); or if mothers receive very low wages (Moore & Driscoll, 1997). Several features of New Hope reduced the likelihood of these negative effects. Although many New Hope participants worked in low status jobs, many of which were probably low in complexity, their employment generated more economic benefits (i.e., earnings supplements, child care and health care subsidies) than would typically be the case for individuals working in low-wage jobs.

Parenting behavior. New Hope was expected to increase adaptive functioning among children partly by improving their home lives. In keeping with the family stress model, with more income, parents' mental health, and in turn, parenting behavior, might improve, leading to higher levels of social and academic competence in children. Adult psychological well-being is strongly linked to both income and emotional support (McLoyd, 1990), and some research with economically disadvantaged single mothers has found a positive association between employment and psychological well-being (Sears & Galambos, 1993). As discussed in a prior section of the chapter, there is also a strong association between parental well-being and positive parenting behaviors (McLoyd, 1990). Taken together, these findings suggest that parents in New Hope might experience improved psychological functioning and in turn, express positive emotions more freely, use more effective family management strategies, and have more positive relationships with their children.

Child care. By providing subsidies for center-based care, the New Hope program made structured child care more accessible to low-income families. Because of the costs of child care, economically disadvantaged families tend to rely on relatives for care, even though they often prefer center-based care (Phillips & Bridgman, 1995; Quint, Bos, & Polit, 1997; Scarr, 1998). Center-based child care often provides more educational opportunities to children and may lead to more advanced cognitive and language development than informal care (Lamb, 1998; NICHD, 2000). The impact of child care on children's development, both social and cognitive, depends largely on the quality of the center. High quality daycare has been shown to buffer against declines in intellectual functioning that are normally associated with high-risk environments (Burchinal, Campbell, Bryant, Wasik, & Ramey, 1997). Because child care subsidies could only be used for licensed care facilities, New Hope was expected to result in higher-quality child care for children.

Child activities. As a consequence of increased family income and increased used of center-based care, children in New Hope were expected to spend more time in organized activities away from home, such as sports, youth clubs, and lessons. Increased income would enhance parents' ability to pay for these activities for their children and center-based child care would provide more opportunities to participate in such activities. In turn, participation in organized activities might have positive impacts on children in New Hope if these activities provided supervision and opportunities for children to explore new interests and participate in learning activities. There is evidence that participation in structured activities allows youth to develop new skills and reduces their involvement in deviant behavior (Task Force on Youth Development and Community Programs, 1992). Research also indicates that participation in formal after-school programs that provide cognitive stimulation is associated with stronger academic achievement among low-income children (Posner & Vandell, 1994).

As shown in Fig. 2, New Hope can be viewed more parsimoniously as a test of two models—the *family stress model* and the *investment model*. The investment model contends that income is associated with children's development because it enables families to invest in the human capital of their children by purchasing materials, experiences, and services that benefit the child's development and well-being (e.g., Linver, Brooks-Gunn, & Kohen, 2002). Whereas the investment model hypothesizes that increases in income produce positive changes in child care and activities and, in turn, positive changes in child functioning, the family stress model posits that increases in income produce positive changes in child functioning through changes in parenting behavior. Below, I briefly summarize the effects of New Hope at three time points—2 years, 5 years, and 8 years after random assignment. For each time point, effects on child functioning are discussed first, followed by effects on children's environments thought to mediate child effects.

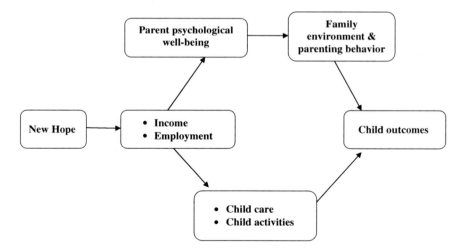

Fig. 2 The New Hope evaluation as a test of the family stress model and the investment model

Two-Year Evaluation

Two years after random assignment, we collected information about the behavioral and psychological functioning of children ages 3–12 years. This age range was chosen to include children in the preschool years and in middle childhood during the 2-year period. There is evidence that family income is especially important during the preschool years (Duncan & Brooks-Gunn, 1997) and the top of this age range coincided with the upper limit for the child care subsidy (Huston et al., 2001).

Impacts on children. In general, New Hope had stronger and more positive impacts on boys than girls. New Hope had positive effects on boys' academic achievement, classroom behavior skills, social behavior, and problem behaviors as reported by teachers (who were unaware of whether the child was in the experimental group or control group). New Hope parents also reported higher levels of positive behaviors for boys than control group parents. In addition, New Hope had positive effects on boys' own expectations for advanced education and occupational aspirations. Boys in New Hope were more likely to expect they that would attend and complete college (6–12 year olds) and aspired to higher prestige managerial and professional occupations (9–12 year olds). There were not corresponding program effects for girls. Indeed, in contrast to the positive effects on boy's behavior, New Hope had significant negative effects on girls' behavior. Teacher reports indicated that New Hope girls, compared to girls in the control sample, showed more externalizing problems (e.g., aggressive behaviors, lack of behavioral control) and required discipline more often (Huston et al., 2001).

It is important to point out that these sex differences in program impacts occurred in the context of more positive scores overall for girls than boys. For example, girls generally were doing better in school and had better study skills than did boys. Additionally, teachers rated girls much lower than they did boys on problem behaviors, and both teachers and parents rated girls higher than boys on positive social behavior. Boys may have been more susceptible to New Hope impacts because their level of functioning at baseline was markedly below that of girls.

Impacts on children's environments. New Hope had effects on the environments of all the children, not just boys. Compared to control group members, program group members reported significantly more quarters of employment, more hours of employment, and more total income over the 2-year period. In addition to boosting family income and parental employment, New Hope increased the amount of time children spent in formal child care programs (compared to preschool and school-aged children in the control group, those in the program group spent almost twice as many months in center-based child care and more than twice as many months in school-based extended day care) and the amount of time children spent in structured activities away from home (children whose parents were in New Hope were significantly more involved in clubs, youth groups, and activities at community centers).

Although program effects on overall formal child care were found for both boys and girls, there were significant sex differences in treatment impacts for extended day care and center-based care. The program-control difference in extended day care was significant for boys, but not for girls, largely because program families used it much more for boys than for girls. On the other hand, although center-based care was used more for both boys and girls in the program group than in the control group, the difference was significantly larger for girls. Although the impact of the program on total structured activity participation did not differ by child sex, there were sex differences in New Hope's impact on participation in clubs and youth groups and going to recreation or community centers. Program-control differences for these outcomes were significant for boys, but not for girls.

This pattern of findings led us to conclude that New Hope had stronger and more positive impacts on boys' academic, behavioral, and psychological functioning than girls' partly because, on the whole, it had stronger effects on boys' proximal environment. Ethnographic interviews among a randomly selected subsample of program and control families, conducted as part of the 2-year follow-up, suggested that parents were especially worried about their sons becoming involved in delinquent activity (Weisner et al., 1999). New Hope's impact on boys' child care experiences and involvement in adult-supervised structured activities probably reflected this worry and program parents' decision to invest resources in their sons to insure that they spent minimal time with unsupervised peers after school (Huston et al., 2001).

Increased family income, greater parental employment, and more time in formal child care programs and in organized activities away from home appear to be implicated in New Hope's impacts on boys' functioning, but parenting did not appear to be a significant mediating pathway. Contrary to our expectations, New Hope did not have consistent or robust impacts on parenting or on parent-child relationships. There were a few favorable impacts on parents' psychological well-being, but they did not translate into more sensitive or effective parenting behavior or improved parent-child relations in the sample overall. For example, parents in New Hope reported greater "hope" (agency and pathways to goals), lower stress, and more social support than control group parents, but they also reported more time pressure. They did not differ from control group parents in terms of worries about finances, self-esteem, mastery, or depressive symptomatology. Despite examining a diverse set of parenting behaviors (e.g., self-reported parental warmth, observed parental warmth, parental control, monitoring), we found no overall effects on parenting as perceived by observers, parents, or children. There were a few positive impacts on parents' relationships with their male children, however. Compared to control group boys, program group boys perceived relations with their parents as more positive and were more likely to think that their parents expected them to attend college. Conversely, girls in New Hope were less likely than control group girls to think that their parents expected them to attend college (Huston et al., 2001).

Five-Year Evaluation

New Hope benefits ended after 3 years. Hence, the 5-year follow-up evaluation indicated whether impacts on children and families persisted, dissipated, or increased 2 years after families left the program.

Impacts on children. Impacts on child functioning at the 5-year follow-up are shown in Figs. 3, 4, and 5, expressed as effect sizes. The effect size is the difference between the program and control group outcomes expressed as a proportion of the

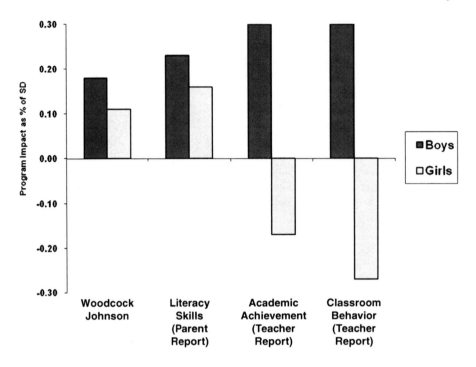

Fig. 3 Impact of New Hope on academic achievement and classroom behavior at 5-year follow-up, by gender

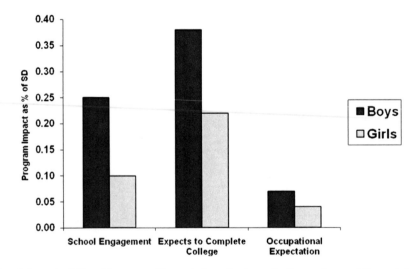

Fig. 4 Impact of New Hope on self-reported academic motivation and expectations at 5-year follow-up, by gender

I

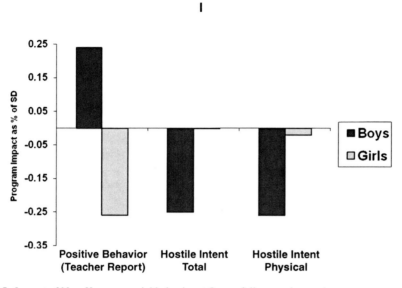

Fig. 5 Impact of New Hope on social behavior at 5-year follow-up, by gender

standard deviation of the outcome for both groups combined. Many of the significant effects found at 24 months were still present 3 years later, although generally, effect sizes had diminished.

Numerous positive impacts were found on indicators of academic achievement, aspirations, and expectations. Teachers still rated boys in New Hope significantly higher on academic achievement than control group boys, but the program had no impact on girls' academic achievement as rated by teachers (Fig. 3). Effects on other indicators of achievement were found for both girls and boys. Children in New Hope scored significantly higher than those in the control group on the Broad Reading component of the Woodcock-Johnson test of achievement. They also received higher overall achievement scores, although the effect was just short of statistical significance. Both male and female children in New Hope scored higher than their peers in the control group, but the effect was stronger for boys. Parents in the program group, compared to those in the control group, reported higher reading and literacy skills among both boys and girls. Unlike the findings at the 2-year follow-up, there were no program effects on occupational expectations for either boys or girls (Huston et al., 2003, 2005). However, boys in New Hope families had higher educational expectations and were more engaged with school than their control group counterparts, but girls did not (Fig. 4).

Teachers continued to rate program boys higher than control boys on classroom behavior skills and positive behavior, but rated program girls lower than control girls (Figs. 3 and 5). In addition, they reported more internalizing problems among New Hope girls than their counterparts. Boys in New Hope families, compared to those in control families, perceived less hostile intent in physical and social vignettes intended to tap aggressive tendencies. However, there were no effects on girls' responses to the stories (Fig. 5).

Impacts on children's environments. The effects on children, taken together, are impressive in light of the fact that most of the economic impacts of New Hope had faded at the 5-year follow-up. New Hope's employment effect as measured by the number of quarters parents were employed annually, while positive, was no longer significant after the first 2 years of the program. Nonetheless, its impact was sufficient to produce a statistically significant increase in the average amount of employment over the entire 5-year period following random assignment (i.e., mean number of quarters employed annually, averaged over 5-year period) (Huston et al., 2003). At the 5-year follow-up, New Hope participants had more stable jobs that paid slightly higher wages than did their control group counterparts, with New Hope participants increasing in average annual income during the entire 5-year period by 7% (Huston et al., 2003).

Similar to the findings 3 years prior, at the 5-year follow-up, there were large differences between the program and control groups in the use of center-based child care, even though child-care benefits had ended. Overall, children in the program group spent significantly more months in center-based child care and in before- and after-school programs (Fig. 6). They also spent significantly fewer months in home-based care than did children from control group families. Among older children (11–16 year olds), program group children spent fewer months in unsupervised care than control group children (Fig. 6).

The impacts on children's involvement in structured activities also carried forth to the 5-year mark. Program group parents reported that their children engaged in

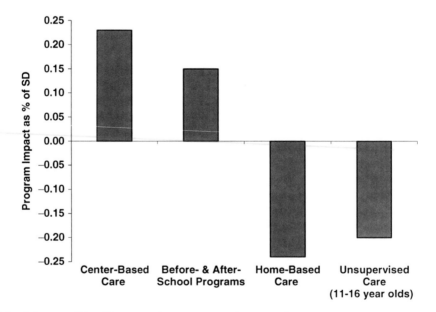

Fig. 6 Impact of New Hope on child care at 5-year follow-up, full sample

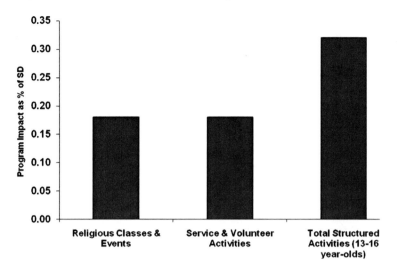

Fig. 7 Impact of New Hope on children's structured activities at 5-year follow-up, full sample

significantly more religious classes and events and more service and volunteer activities than did control group children. For adolescents (13–16 year olds), New Hope led to higher levels of participation in a composite score for structured activities (i.e., lessons, organized sports, clubs and youth groups, religious activities and activities at recreational and community centers) (Fig. 7).

Effects on parents' psychological well-being were weaker than those found at the 2-year follow-up, but had not faded completely. Parents in New Hope reported fewer depressive symptoms than did parents in the control group. This impact, however, did not result in more positive parenting or parent-child relations. There were no overall impacts on any of the four aggregate measures of parenting (effective child management, warm and structured parenting, positive parent-child relations, and negative parent-child relations). Some impacts for specific gender and age groups were found, but they were sparse and scattered (Huston et al., 2005).

Eight-Year Evaluation

The 8-year evaluation, conducted when youth were ages 9–19, included categories of dependent variables similar to those in the two prior follow-ups (e.g., social behavior, academic achievement and motivation) as well as measures of youth's future orientation (i.e., attitudes and expectancies about work, involvement in employment and career preparation activities) and employment experiences (e.g., probability of employment, duration and intensity of employment, employment earnings). We gave special attention to the latter two domains for several reasons. First, as discussed below, they encompass important developmental markers during mid to late adolescence. Second, youth's future orientation and employment experiences are highly relevant to the developmental goals that youth development leaders advocate (e.g., preparation for a lifetime of meaningful work), and to specific competencies that these leaders regard as necessary for a healthy and productive adulthood (e.g., awareness and understanding of life options, knowledge of steps needed to make educational and occupational choices, understanding the value and purpose of work and family) (Roth, Murray, Brooks-Gunn, & Foster, 1999). Third, evidence that New Hope had positive impacts on these outcomes may signal the program's potential for breaking the cycle of poverty and facilitating intergenerational mobility. Before summarizing the findings for all of the outcome variables, I discuss why future orientation and employment experiences are important for low-income youth and the bases on which we expected New Hope to influence these outcomes.

Future orientation. Among lower SES adolescents, planning for the future predicts upward social mobility in adulthood (Clausen, 1991). Moreover, positive future orientation among adolescents is associated with lower risk of several problematic behaviors linked to low-income status (e.g., substance abuse, delinquency, adolescent pregnancy) (Murray, 1996; Wyman et al., 1992). There is also evidence linking positive future orientation and expectations to higher levels of well-being among disadvantaged and at-risk adolescent populations, including better socioemotional and school adjustment (Wyman, Cowen, Work, & Kerley, 1993), greater feelings of efficacy and responsibility for one's life and decisions (Kerpelman & Mosher, 2004), and fewer conduct problems (Quinton, Pickles, Maughan, & Rutter, 1993).

There were several reasons to expect that New Hope would lead to more positive future orientations. First, New Hope increased children's involvement in before- and after-school programs and adult-supervised structured activities (Huston et al., 2005) and this impact might boost children's psychological well-being. Organized activities away from home afford opportunities to develop skills, interests, and social relationships with peers, as well as opportunities to develop mentoring relationships with caring adults. In low-income and ethnic minority youth, mentoring relationships are associated with greater self-confidence and optimism, higher educational achievement and the absence of a gap between educational aspirations and expectations (Hellenga, Aber, & Rhodes, 2002; Sanchez, Esparza, & Colon, 2008). There is also evidence that youth who participate in organized out-of-school activities have higher levels of achievement, higher school motivation, and greater social competence than do nonparticipants (Mahoney, Larson, & Eccles, 2005), outcomes that may in turn, enhance optimism about the future.

Second, it was plausible that New Hope would positively affect children's future orientation indirectly through its effects on parents' earnings and income. Recall that at the 5-year follow-up, New Hope participants had more stable jobs that paid slightly higher wages than did their control group counterparts. New Hope also significantly reduced family-level poverty over the 5-year period following random assignment, and the effects were equally strong in both the early years (1–3) and the later years (4–5) (Huston et al., 2003). These economic outcomes, together, might render New Hope parents stronger role models of employment whose working lives exemplified more prominently the value and rewards of employment. Third, more direct effects of parents' improved economic status were also plausible. Prior research indicates that adolescents are more optimistic about their economic and occupational futures if their parents are employed (Quane & Rankin, 1998), if they perceive their families as experiencing less financial strain (Flanagan, 1990; Larson, 1984; McLoyd & Jozefowicz, 1996), and if they perceive their parents as having more favorable work experiences (Neblett & Cortina, 2006).

Impacts on future orientation were expected to be larger for boys than girls because of prior gender differences in New Hope's impact on children's educational expectations. Higher expectations might translate into greater optimism about the future among program group boys, given evidence that educational expectations predict occupational expectations and mediate links between socioeconomic status and youth's occupational expectations (Cook et al., 1996).

Adolescent employment experiences. Within the general adolescent population, whether employment is linked to problematic functioning (e.g., delinquency, truncated schooling, lower school performance) or positive adjustment is conditional on myriad factors, including the number of hours worked, type of job (typical teenage jobs vs. adult jobs), and the adolescent's previous level of academic achievement, age, gender, and social class (see Zimmer-Gembeck & Mortimer, 2006 for a review). However, the few existing studies of employment among low-income adolescents, and among ethnic minority adolescents, generally point to beneficial effects and few negative effects (Bauermeister, Zimmerman, Barnett, & Caldwell, 2007; Johnson, 2004).

Low-income African American youth who enter the workforce earlier are more likely to complete high school than peers who enter the workforce later during adolescence, and low SES males with poor school performance appear to benefit from work experience by improving their prospects for future employment (Entwisle, Alexander, & Olson, 2000; Leventhal, Graber, & Brooks-Gunn, 2001). Ethnographic work also points to beneficial effects, suggesting that employment provides low-income youth structured supports that foster continued education and buttress motivation to attain higher levels of schooling (Newman, 1999). There is evidence that average number of hours worked per week during adolescence is positively correlated with earnings during young adulthood (mid to late 20's), irrespective of social class (Ruhm, 1997), although some studies have not replicated this finding (e.g., Light, 1995).

Perhaps the relation between employment and positive adjustment is stronger and more consistent for low-income adolescents than economically advantaged adolescents because of class-related differences in the meaning and functions of adolescent employment. For economically advantaged adolescents, employment during high school typically is a source of pocket money for leisure spending and has little bearing on post-high school employment outcomes or college attendance. For poor or near poor students—most of whom lack the means to go to college—employment during high school may not only help meet family needs, but also may forecast more favorable post-high school employment outcomes as a result of the practical skills and expanded social networks it affords (Entwisle et al., 2000; Newman, 1999; Ruhm, 1997). Taken as a whole, extant research justifies viewing adolescent employment among low-income youth as a developmental asset, rather than a risk factor, especially if it is moderate in intensity (i.e., <20 hr/week).

We expected New Hope to increase the probability, duration, and intensity of employment and increase employment earnings among boys because at the 5-year follow-up, it positively affected several of the psychological and behavioral correlates of youth employment (i.e., school achievement, school engagement, social competence). New Hope also might increase employment among adolescents if their parents' stronger attachment to the labor market afforded them family connections to jobs.

Impacts on children. Although most of the earlier positive effects on social behavior, achievement, and achievement motivation had dissipated, a few effects remained and importantly, there was no evidence of reversal or negative long-term impacts on children. In addition, some effects that held for only boys in prior follow-ups were evident for the full sample. Five years after the program ended, there were no significant effects on any teacher-reported scales of social behavior, but program parents rated their children higher than did control group parents on positive social behavior (an aggregate score composed of subscales measuring social competence, compliance, and autonomy) and lower on such internalizing behavior problems as sadness and social withdrawal (Huston et al., 2008, 2009). Moreover, New Hope had significant positive impacts on youth's overall progress in school (e.g., less grade retention, lower enrollment in special education) and their school engagement, although its impact on most measures of educational achievement had faded. Some effects held only for boys. Boys in New Hope scored higher on the Woodcock-Johnson Broad Reading scale, held higher expectancies for performing well in English, and were more likely to expect to attend and graduate from college than control group boys (Huston et al., 2009).

We found support for several of our hypotheses about future orientation, but only among boys (McLoyd, Kaplan, & Purtell, in press). Boys in program group families held less cynical attitudes about work than those in control group families. For example, they were less likely to agree with the statements "If I had the chance, I would go through life without ever working," "Workers are entitled to call in sick when they don't feel like working," and "Most people today are stuck in dead end, go-nowhere jobs." In addition, New Hope boys were less pessimistic about their economic futures (e.g., lower expectations of losing a job as an adult or encountering difficulty finding a good job) and more involved in employment and career preparation activities (e.g., talked with adults outside of school about careers, work, and what they will do after high school; got instruction or counseling on how to find a job; studied in class about different kinds of jobs and requirements for the jobs) than boys in control group families (Fig. 8). These effects were most pronounced among African American boys, with very few effects found for European American and Hispanic boys. These ethnic differences in New Hope's impact are likely due in part to insufficient statistical power to detect effects on European American and Hispanic boys. The samples of Hispanic and European American boys were substantially smaller than the sample of African American boys ($n = 268$, 104, and 69 for African American, Hispanic, and European American boys, respectively).

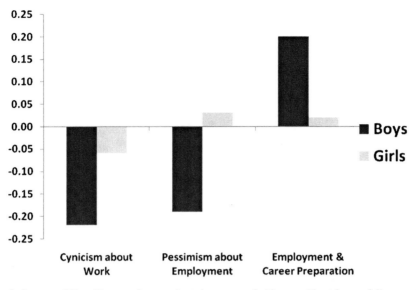

Fig. 8 Impact of New Hope on future orientation among 9–19 year olds at 8-year follow-up, by gender

Gender differences also existed in impacts on employment experiences among 12–19 year olds. Boys in program group families worked at higher levels of intensity (greater number of hours per week) during the school year than boys in control group families, whereas New Hope had no impact on girls' employment experiences (Fig. 9). Strong ethnic differences were also found. African American youth in

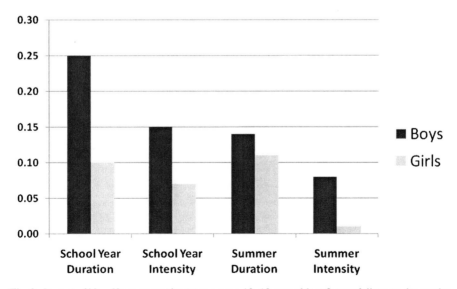

Fig. 9 Impact of New Hope on employment among 12–19 year olds at 8-year follow-up, by gender

program families worked for longer periods of time during the summer months and during the school year, worked at higher levels of intensity, and earned more money than their counterparts in control families. No effects were found for Hispanic or European American youth (McLoyd et al., in press).

Impacts on children's environments. Comparisons of the average employment and earnings of parents in New Hope and control group parents showed no overall differences 5 years after the end of the program (Duncan et al., 2008). However, impacts on children's activities persisted, although they were diminished. Based on parental reports, New Hope children continued to participate in more organized out-of-school activities, averaging across five activities (lessons, organized sports, clubs and youth groups, religious classes and events, activities at recreation or community centers), as compared with control group children. When activities were analyzed separately, the impact held only for religious activities. New Hope youth also reported spending more time in volunteer and service activities. There were no impacts on parents' psychological well-being. Parents in New Hope reported more effective child management than control group parents—that is, they used less punishment, felt less parenting stress, and felt they had better control of their children (Huston et al., 2008), but overall there were few impacts on parenting behavior.

Interpreting the New Hope Findings

Although 2 and 5 years after random assignment, New Hope produced higher levels of psychological well-being among parents, it had surprisingly few impacts on parenting behavior and parent-child relations, suggesting that proximal parenting behavior was *not* a pathway through which New Hope influenced child well-being. Rather, the overall pattern of findings point strongly and consistently to formal child care and children's involvement in organized activities—out-of-home explanations—for New Hope's impact. In this regard, the findings are more compatible with the investment model (Linver et al., 2002), as these experiences and services were purchased partly with subsidies when New Hope was in operation and perhaps entirely by parents after New Hope ended.

It is surprising that the findings lend little support for the family stress model, given the robust support that correlational research has found for this model. Although it is possible that the brief self-report measures of parenting were insufficiently sensitive to detect treatment effects, the findings nonetheless raise questions about whether correlational research has overestimated the influence of proximal parenting behavior as a mediator of the link between income and children's socioemotional and academic functioning. The effects of New Hope on child outcomes are particularly persuasive because many effects persisted and because effects appeared on measures obtained from multiple sources. Measures obtained from parents, who were the most likely to be affected by their knowledge of the New Hope treatment and the evaluation design, showed fewer treatment differences than did measures completed by teachers (who were unaware of whether the child was the experimental group or control group) and children.

The fact that many impacts on children's functioning were evident long after the program ended suggests that New Hope created positive shifts in children's developmental trajectories. Our conclusion that formal child care, before- and after-school programs, and organized out-of-school activities played major roles in promoting these positive shifts is consistent with a growing body of evidence that how children spend their time has important developmental consequences (Larson, 2000). Spending time in organized activities provides opportunities for youth to develop interpersonal and academic skills and has been linked to numerous positive outcomes such as diminished delinquency and higher academic achievement (Larson, 2000; Mahoney et al., 2005). Research also indicates that center-based care, on average, is more likely than home-based care to enhance cognitive, academic, and social skills (Lamb, 1998; Loeb, Fuller, Kagan, & Carrol, 2004). It is also significant that well after the New Hope child care subsidy ended, children in New Hope families continued to spend significantly more time than control group children in formal center-based care and before- and after-school programs. The most likely explanation for these effects is that New Hope parents came to value organized programs and learned how to access public and private resources available to them (Huston et al., 2003).

New Hope's impact on children's socioemotional adjustment, achievement, and involvement in organized activities can be framed more broadly in terms of Lareau's (2003) concept of "concerted cultivation." This concept refers to a child-rearing approach in which parents actively foster and assess children's talents, opinions, and skills and provide children with multiple leisure activities that adults orchestrate and supervise. Lareau's research suggests that elements of "concerted cultivation" are highly salient in middle-class families, whereas working-class and low-income parents are likely to rely on "the accomplishment of natural growth" as a primary child-rearing strategy. This class differential likely reflects differences in financial resources with which to provide children growth-enhancing opportunities, disparities in available time to engage in activities with children, and differing perspectives on how parents should be involved in their child's schooling and activities. By increasing income, promoting more stable employment, and providing options for structured child care, New Hope may have increased low-income children's opportunities for "concerted cultivation."

Although there are costs and benefits to both child-rearing strategies, one of the most significant benefits of concerted cultivation for low-income children may be the promotion of skills and sensibilities that foster positive experiences outside of the family such as school and work settings. Lareau's (2003) in-depth ethnographies indicate that children who participated in extra-curricular activities learned new skills and behaviors that were useful in other contexts. For example, they learned appropriate ways to present themselves and to interact with non-family members. In addition, scholars suggest that within the context of organized activities, children develop relationships with other adults who may serve as role models and mentors. As a consequence, they may begin to develop a trust of institutions beyond their family. These experiences help youth to understand what is expected of them in school, handle authority in appropriate ways, and maintain positive social relations with classmates. In addition, they tend to nurture initiative, which fosters success in academic pursuits (Mahoney et al., 2005).

Lareau's work focuses on children, but the concepts and processes described in her work are applicable to adolescents as well. Because of the increased need for adult guidance in relation to major decisions pondered during adolescence, such as post-high training and education and choosing a career, connections to responsible, caring adults and institutions increase the likelihood of positive adolescent development (Jarrett, 1995). Thus, increased experiences of "concerted cultivation" may be a possible path to successful development for low-income youth.

Gender differences. A surprising and important outcome of New Hope is the striking gender differences in the impacts on children. To understand why the program's positive impacts were largely limited to boys, a number of post-hoc hypotheses were explored. We explored the possibility that the increase in maternal employment led to more household chores and child care responsibilities for daughters than sons in the program, but found no evidence to support this hypothesis. We also found no support for the idea that New Hope girls became more independent or assertive as a result of their parents' involvement in work, and hence, were perceived by teachers as having more externalizing problems (Huston et al., 2005).

As indicated previously, the gender disparities in New Hope's impact on child functioning appear to be driven largely by gender differences in the program's impact on children's environment. In particular, New Hope may have had stronger and more positive impacts on boys' academic, behavioral, and psychological functioning than girls partly because it increased boys', but not girls' participation in before- and after-school programs, clubs, youth groups, and activities at recreational and community centers. These experiences and the academic and social competencies that New Hope conferred to program boys at the 2- and 5-year follow-ups may account for the positive effects of New Hope on boys' attitudes about work and employment experiences at the 8-year follow-up. This developmental continuity is quite plausible given evidence that higher school achievement and fewer problem behaviors predict higher levels of employment among low-income youth. Wilson's (1996) seminal study of urban employment indicates that poor reading and math skills are significant contributors to the failure of low-income youth to find employment. The effects of New Hope on boys' future orientation and employment experiences also could have resulted from advantages accrued during the 3-year benefit period, which altered boys' trajectories and led to an upward spiral. Boys' better school performance as rated by teachers at the 2-year evaluation, for example, could have led to experiences of success and feelings of efficacy and optimism that were self-perpetuating.

It bears repeating that the strong pattern of sex differences in the impact of the New Hope program should be evaluated in light of the absolute differences between girls and boys on most of the indicators of child functioning. Girls generally showed more positive behaviors, exhibited fewer problem behaviors, and had higher levels of school performance and more positive orientations to the future than did boys. In general, New Hope brought boys' level of functioning closer to the typical levels for girls in both the program and control group.

Ethnic differences. Five years after the program ended, New Hope positively impacted the employment experiences of African American youth, but not Hispanics and Whites. There is little to suggest that New Hope's impact on adolescent employment put African American youth at developmental risk. Employed adolescents typically worked well below 20 hr/week, even those who were at the higher end of the distribution in work hours. It is high levels of work intensity (i.e., >20 hr/week) that has been most consistently linked to negative outcomes (e.g., delinquent behavior) (Zimmer-Gembeck & Mortimer, 2006).

Impacts on future orientation were pronounced among African American males, a group whose struggles in the labor market are especially acute. African American and Latino boys have the highest unemployment rates among youth (Bureau of Labor Statistics, 2000) and these rates persist into adulthood (Edelman, Holzer, & Offner, 2006). By reducing African American boys' cynicism about work and pessimism about future employment, and increasing their career preparation, New Hope may enhance their longer-term engagement in the labor market and ultimately, their chances of securing stable jobs with good wages. Wilson's (1996) work clearly shows that a primary reason inner city employers prefer to hire African American females to African American males is their more positive work-related attitudes.

Implications for Policy

The total cost of New Hope was relatively high (approximately $18,000 per CFS family in 2005 dollars), but if the positive effects of New Hope on child functioning ultimately result in less crime, less incarceration, and less welfare use, the savings may exceed program costs several times over (Duncan et al., 2007). Due to funding constraints, eligibility for New Hope benefits was limited to 3 years. However, designers of New Hope envisioned it as a model for a work support program that would be permanently available to all low-income workers (Bos et al., 1999). The existence of such a program does not mean that everyone would receive supports for a lifetime (e.g., over time, the incomes of some would rise above the income eligibility limit; some of the employed would receive health insurance through their employers; individuals would not meet the work requirement all the time, etc.) (Duncan et al., 2007).

Federal and state policies enacted during the 1990s to strengthen work supports for low-income families resemble, but in many ways fall short of replicating, the benefits that New Hope offered. The Earned Income Tax Credit (EITC), essentially an earnings-supplement program for low-income workers, was greatly expanded in the 1990s and more recently with the passage of the American Recovery and Reinvestment Act of 2009. Families with two or more children are eligible for a maximum of $4,400 annually (Berlin, 2007; H.R.1., 2009). This is a progressive trend in light of the effects of New Hope and evidence that increases in income have much stronger impacts on cognitive functioning among children in families with incomes below or near the poverty line than among children in middle-class or affluent families (Duncan & Brooks-Gunn, 1997; Smith, Brooks-Gunn, &

Klebanov, 1997). Both the EITC and New Hope's earnings supplement were significant sources of income for families in New Hope. However, New Hope's earnings supplement differed from the EITC in an important way. Because EITC benefits are tied to earnings, individuals can receive the EITC for part-time work. This may provide an incentive for higher-wage workers to cut hours in order to receive maximum benefits (Duncan et al., 2007). Making earnings supplements conditional on full-time work, while insuring that the total incomes of full-time workers increased with earnings, as New Hope did, likely would encourage greater amounts of employment, increase stable employment, and importantly, increase family income.

Safe, reliable child care is essential to working parents, but its high cost is especially challenging for low-income families. When low-income working families pay for child care, they purchase less expensive care than higher-income families, but pay a much larger share of their income for it (Greenberg, 2007). The largest percentage of New Hope program costs over the 3-year eligibility period came from child care subsidies (38%, followed by case management and administration of benefits at 23%) and it is indeed in the area of child care assistance that the largest disparity exists between New Hope benefits and existing policies. New Hope guaranteed child care subsidies to full-time employed parents of children under age 13 and enabled parents to choose from a range of options because it paid most of the cost. Subsidized child care had to be provided in state-licensed or county certified homes or child care centers. Subsidies were paid directly to child care providers on a monthly basis which had the advantage that families did not have to wait for reimbursement of child care costs (Huston et al., 2003).

Federal child care policy consists of two principal components—a tax credit that goes primarily to middle- and upper-income families and block grant funding to states to help low-income working families with child care costs (Greenberg, 2007). In the mid-2000s, block grant funding declined and fewer states had excess TANF funds to pay for child care. Many low-income families do not receive child care assistance due to long waiting lists and lack of knowledge about assistance programs. In 2004, nearly half of the states either had a waiting list for subsidized child care or had closed enrollment and were not even maintaining a waiting list (Duncan et al., 2007). Clearly, policies that more effectively address the child care needs of low-income working parents are sorely needed. Our findings, together with evidence that center-based care, on average, is more likely than home-based care to enhance cognitive, academic, and social skills, suggest that children will benefit from policies that significantly expand child care subsidies for low-income working families and increase the availability of high-quality center-based child care, after-school care, and opportunities for supervised, structured activities.

Beyond New Hope: Syntheses of the Effects of Employment-Based Welfare and Anti-poverty Policies

The New Hope Program is one example of a work-based anti-poverty intervention, but numerous others have been implemented. Findings from any single program with an income supplement such as New Hope require tenuous statements about the effects of income per se because benefits and services within a program typically are offered as a package, making it impossible to identify the separate effects of different components of the program. However, consideration of findings across multiple programs whose common feature is income supplements (with a mixture of other program services) increases confidence in the causal effects of income supplements.

Morris and colleagues (Morris et al., 2001) examined the findings from five large-scale studies, including the New Hope evaluation, that together assessed the effects on preschoolers and elementary school-age children of 11 different employment-based welfare and antipoverty programs aimed primarily at single parent families. All of the studies used a treatment-control randomized research design. Morris et al. found that programs such as New Hope that included earning supplements increased both parental employment and income. Moreover, these programs had modest, positive effects on a range of child behaviors. All of these programs had overall positive effects on children's school achievement (by approximately 10–15%, as compared to children in the control groups), and some also reduced behavior problems, increased positive social behavior, and/or improved children's overall health. Importantly, none of the programs had overall negative impacts on children's behaviors. Some programs, such as New Hope, had effects primarily on boys, while others had stronger effects for girls. There was no clear pattern of gender differences when looking across different experiments. In contrast, Morris and her colleagues (2001) found that programs with mandatory employment services (i.e., programs in which cash welfare benefits were contingent on education, training, or immediate job search) successfully increased parental employment rates and reduced welfare receipt, but generally left family income unchanged because participants lost welfare benefits as their earnings increased. Furthermore, these programs had few effects on children, and the effects found were mixed in direction.

Although all of the earnings supplement programs increased employment and income, no one mechanism appeared to be responsible for the beneficial effects of these programs on children. None of the outcomes considered to be possible mediators of effects (i.e., parental well-being, parenting behavior, family relations, child care) was affected across all of programs For example, some programs improved parents' psychological functioning (e.g., fewer symptoms of depression, less parental stress, greater sense of agency), but others did not. Likewise, whereas some programs increased the use of formal and stable child care and children's participation in after-school activities, others had no impact on these outcomes. In general, none of the experiments had strong, consistent impacts on parenting behavior (Morris et al., 2001).

Gennetian and colleagues (2004) conducted a synthesis of research focusing on children who were *adolescents* (ages 10–16) when their parents began participating in the employment-based welfare and antipoverty programs. Their findings are strikingly different from those that emerged from Morris et al.'s synthesis focusing on children who were preschoolers and elementary school students when their parents began participating in the program. In particular, Gennetian et al. found negative impacts on adolescents' educational achievement across the board, regardless of whether the program provided earnings supplements, mandated employment services, or imposed time limits. The impacts were somewhat small, but still significant. Programs with mandatory employment increased use of special education services for an emotional, physical, or mental condition, whereas programs with earnings benefits, which had positive impacts on younger children, increased adolescent dropout rates. Furthermore, programs with time limits reduced school performance. Gennetian et al.'s synthesis suggests that New Hope's impacts might have been different if most children had been in the midst of adolescence during the time their families participated in the program.

It is not altogether clear why adolescents, on average, fared less well than preschool and elementary school-age children under these experimental programs, but there is some suggestion that the programs tended to change adolescents' ecologies in ways that were largely incompatible with their developmental needs, whereas the reverse seemed true for preschoolers and elementary school-age children. For example, Gennetian et al.(2004) found some tentative evidence that these programs tended to increase intensive adolescent employment, decrease adult supervision, and increase domestic responsibilities (e.g., sibling care)—all factors that have the potential to impose time pressures that interfere with adolescents' engagement in school and completion of homework. Detrimental impacts on adolescents were stronger for those adolescents who had a younger sibling, lending support to the idea that increases in domestic responsibilities in response to parental employment can negatively affect adolescents' academic and psychological functioning. In contrast, for preschool and school-age children, several of these programs led to increases in the amount of time they spent in formal child care and organized before- and after-school activities—both of which have been linked to enhanced cognitive, academic, and social functioning (Gennetian et al., 2004; Morris et al., 2001).

Directions for Future Research

In this section, I offer several recommendations for increasing our understanding of processes influencing socioemotional adjustment in economically disadvantaged youth.

Extend the Search for Mediating and Moderating Processes

Contrary to the family stress model, changes in parenting behavior did not emerge as prominent or core mediators of the experimental effects of New Hope or other employment-based welfare and antipoverty experiments on children's socioemotional functioning or school achievement. Rather, these studies suggest that increases in family income enhanced child functioning less through changes in parenting behavior and home environment and more through changes in out-of-home experiences. Taken as a whole, these studies challenge poverty researchers conducting correlational field studies to expand the search for mediating processes beyond the home and family context and to give special attention to extrafamilial factors that can be readily regulated through public policy.

Psychologists have been criticized for their persistent attention to parental behavior as a mediator of the relation between poverty and children's socioemotional and cognitive functioning, while ignoring the developmental and psychological significance of the overwhelming array of aversive physical conditions that surround poor children (Evans, 2004). Researchers are beginning to redress the lack of attention to the latter issue, but in general, psychologists have given short shrift to forces outside the immediate household or family (with the exception of deviant peers) as potential mediators of links between poverty and children's development. A fuller understanding of the pathways through which poverty and socioeconomic disadvantage affects children requires attention to the multiple ecological contexts within which children are embedded.

In this regard, we need research that clarifies the extent to which chronic poverty and socioeconomic disadvantage adversely affect children's mental health, school achievement, and other areas of functioning by increasing their exposure to demeaning, humiliating, and otherwise negative treatment precipitated by the stigmas of poverty and socioeconomic disadvantage (e.g., Glasgow, 1981; Gouldner, 1978; MacLeod, 1987). Relative to earlier developmental periods, adolescence is distinguished by increased salience of peers and greater exposure to the media (Steinberg & Silk, 2002)—trends likely to increase the prevalence and psychological consequences of social evaluation processes. As a result of cognitive growth, adolescence also brings increased awareness of the social meaning of being poor in a stratified society with high levels of economic inequality (Wiltfang & Scarbecz, 1990), and this awareness often prompts efforts to mask one's disadvantage.

A prosaic, yet poignant, example is displayed during lunch periods in schools across the country. Unlike elementary school children, middle-school children have an aversion to subsidized lunches provided in schools because they comprehend the stigma attached to this subsidy. Because of this increased awareness, combined with heightened sensitivity to peer evaluations during adolescence, the percentage of eligible students who take advantage of federally subsidized meal programs in schools plummets when children reach middle-school. Many middle-school students who are poor, if they do not bring lunches from home, decide to go hungry rather than be seen with a subsidized meal. As one student said, lunchtime "is the best time to impress your peers" and being seen with a subsidized meal "lowers your status" (Pogash, 2008, p. 1). Adolescents who are poor or from socioeconomically disadvantaged backgrounds may be hampered in the use of self-protective strategies found among members of other stigmatized groups (e.g., physically handicapped) because of low levels of class consciousness (in contrast to high levels of race consciousness) and widespread endorsement of individualistic explanations of poverty and socioeconomic disadvantage (Crocker & Major, 1989). The rich empirical literature on stigma provides fertile ground to investigate these issues, as well as ways teachers and other societal agents can blunt stigma and its potential negative psychological effects on low-income children.

Neurobiological models and studies promise to expand our understanding of the pathways through which exposure to chronic stressors linked to poverty impacts adolescent mental health. Scholars working in this area hypothesize, for example, that chronic stressors dysregulate physiological stress response systems, putting adolescents at higher risk of poor decision-making and its consequences (e.g., substance abuse), psychosocial maladjustment, and physical health problems (Bar-On, Tranel, Denburg, & Bechara, 2003; Sinha, 2001). Early work lends preliminary support for some of these hypotheses, although much more work will be required to adequately test them and determine the generalizability of various processes (e.g., Fishbein, Herman-Stahl, & Eldreth, 2006; Sinha, 2001). Research about brain development during adolescence, links between this development and behavior, and the neurobiological effects of poverty-related stress on the developing brain is also likely to significantly advance our understanding of the pathways through which poverty affects mental health. It may also illuminate the extent to which timing of poverty effects found in previous research (e.g., Duncan & Brooks-Gunn, 1997) are biologically-based and, in turn, aid in the design of more efficient and potent prevention programs. Given the complexities and multifaceted nature of these issues, and the different methods that will be required to address them adequately, interdisciplinary research collaborations and research training that crosses disciplinary boundaries seem essential.

Document Determinants and Mediating Effects of Participation in Organized Extracurricular Activities

There is growing evidence that participation in extracurricular activities promotes positive development and that low-income children may experience greater benefits from these activities than adolescents from more economically advantaged backgrounds (e.g., Mahoney et al., 2005). In light of these findings, it is important to identify factors that influence low-income children's participation in extracurricular activities and find ways to encourage and expand participation. More work is needed to understand the processes through which low-income children benefit from extracurricular activities and to determine the types and characteristics of activities that best promote socioemotional and academic competence in these children. Testing the effects of extracurricular participation in a random assignment experimental design is an attractive and highly feasible strategy to address the problems of selection bias.

Identify Resilience Processes in the Context of Chronic Economic Disadvantage

Many healthy and productive adults grew up in poverty. Nonetheless, research on positive adaptation in the context of economic disadvantage and protective processes that mitigate negative outcomes among economically disadvantaged children and adolescents is extremely limited. More work has focused on resilience in the face of specific stressors (e.g., parental alcoholism, child maltreatment, and maternal depression) than resilience in the context of economic disadvantage. Poverty and low-income status are risk factors that are strongly associated with a highly diverse combination of other risk factors. This reality does not preclude examination of protective processes that mitigate the effects of poverty and the cumulative risks associated with poverty. Indeed, scholars have argued that focusing on a single risk factor does not address the reality of most children's lives and that "to truly appreciate the determinants of competence requires attention to the broad constellation of ecological factors in which these individuals and families are embedded" (Sameroff, Gutman, & Peck, 2003, p. 338).

What factors might account for the paucity of research on positive adaptation in the context of socioeconomic disadvantage? Yoshikawa and Seidman (2000) posit two main reasons for this state of affairs in research on adolescents—the disproportionate attention paid to problem behaviors and the idea that competence among low-income adolescents is incompatible with some prominent developmental theories. Research on adolescents has traditionally focused heavily on antisocial and problem behaviors (Furstenberg, 2000), especially when the adolescents in question are poor or from low SES backgrounds. Domains in which adolescents may be highly functional despite difficult circumstances have largely been overlooked (Burton, Obeidallah, & Allison, 1996). Even studies of resilience have tended not to center on positive development, but rather on whether or not problem behaviors exist (Mahoney & Bergman, 2002; Yoshikawa & Seidman, 2000).

Others have raised the possibility that the capacity of positive individual, family, or community factors to either mitigate risks or foster positive outcomes may be compromised under circumstances of extremely high risk (Li, Nussbaum, & Richards, 2007; Luthar, Cicchetti, & Becker, 2000). Still others have argued that some poor and low SES children are growing up in circumstances so dire that positive outcomes are highly unlikely (Cauce, Stewart, Rodriguez, Cochran, & Ginzler, 2003). Because the research literature on children living under conditions of chronic economic hardship has given so little attention to positive adaptation or competence, in general, it is unclear which protective factors are overwhelmed under certain circumstances and which positive outcomes are more common than others. Both policy and theoretical considerations warrant vigorous, systematic efforts to identify and understand protective processes that mitigate negative outcomes among economically disadvantaged children.

References

Bar-On, R., Tranel, D., Denburg, N. L., & Bechara, A. (2003). Exploring the neurological substrate of emotional and social intelligence. *Brain, 126,* 1790–1800.

Bauermeister, J. A., Zimmerman, M. A., Barnett, T. E., & Caldwell, C. H. (2007). Working in high school and adaptation in the transition to young adulthood among African American youth. *Journal of Youth and Adolescence, 36,* 877–890.

Belle, D. (1982). Social ties and social support. In D. Belle (Ed.), *Lives in stress: Women and depression* (pp. 133–144). Beverly Hills, CA: Sage.

Berlin, G. (2007). Rewarding the work of individuals: A counterintuitive approach to reducing poverty and strengthening families. *The Future of Children, 27,* 17–42.

Blank, S. W., & Blum, B. (1997). A brief history of work expectations for welfare mothers. *The Future of Children, 7*(1), 28–38.

Bolger, K. E., Patterson, C. J., & Thompson, W. W. (1995). Psychosocial adjustment among children experiencing persistent and intermittent family economic hardship. *Child Development, 66*(4), 1107–1129.

Bos, J. M., Huston, A. C., Granger, R. C., Duncan, G. J., Brock, T. W., & McLoyd, V. C. (1999). *New Hope for people with low incomes: Two-year results of a program to reduce poverty and reform welfare.* New York: Manpower Demonstration Research Corporation.

Brody, G. H., & Flor, D. (1998). Maternal resources, parenting practices, and child competence in rural, single-parent African American families. *Child Development, 69,* 803–816.

Brody, G. H., Stoneman, Z., & Flor, D. (1995). Linking family processes and academic competence among rural African American youths. *Journal of Marriage and the Family, 57,* 567–579.

Brody, G. H., Stoneman, Z., Flor, D., McCrary, C., Hastings, L., & Conyers, O. (1994). Financial resources, parent psychological functioning, parent co-caregiving, and early adolescent competence in rural two-parent African American families. *Child Development, 65,* 590–605.

Brody, G., Stoneman, Z., Flor, D., McCrary, C., Hastings, L., & Conyers, O. (1994). Financial resources, parent psychological functioning, parent co-caregiving, and early adolescent competence in rural two-parent African-American families. *Child Development, 65,* 590–605.

Bronfenbrenner, U., & Ceci, S. J. (1994). Nature-nurture reconceptualized in developmental perspective: A bioecological model. *Psychology Reviews, 101,* 568–586.

Brooks-Gunn, J., & Furstenberg, F. F. (1989). Adolescent sexual behavior. *American Psychologist, 44,* 249–257.

Burchinal, M. R., Campbell, F. A., Bryant, D. M., Wasik, B. H., & Ramey, C. T. (1997). Early intervention and mediating processes in cognitive performance of children in low-income African American families. *Child Development, 68,* 935–954.

Bureau of Labor Statistics. (2000). *Report on the youth labor force.* Washington, DC: U.S. Department of Labor.

Burton, L. M., Obeidallah, D. A., & Allison, K. (1996). Ethnographic insights on social context and adolescent development among inner-city African American teens. In R. Jessor, A. Colby, & R. A. Shweder (Eds.), *Ethnography and human development: Context and meaning in social inquiry* (pp. 395–418). Chicago: University of Chicago Press.

Campbell, K. E., & Lee, B. A. (1992). Sources of personal neighbor networks: Social integration, need, or time? *Social Forces, 70,* 1077–1100.

Capaldi, D. M., Pears, K. C., Patterson, G. R., & Owen, L. D. (2003). Continuity of parenting practices across generations in an at-risk sample: A prospective comparison of direct and mediated associations. *Journal of Abnormal Child Psychology, 31*(2), 127–142.

Cauce, A. M., Stewart, A., Rodriguez, M. D., Cochran, M., & Ginzler, J. (2003). Overcoming the odds? Adolescent development in the context of urban poverty. In S. S. Luthar (Ed.), *Resilience and vulnerability: Adaptation in the context of childhood adversities* (pp. 343–363). New York: Cambridge University Press.

Ceballo, R., & McLoyd, V. C. (2002). Social support and parenting in poor, dangerous neighborhoods. *Child Development, 73,* 1310–1321.

Cherry, F. F., & Eaton, E. L. (1977). Physical and cognitive development in children of low-income mothers working in the child's early years. *Child Development, 48,* 158–166.

Clausen, J. S. (1991). Adolescent competence and the shaping of the life course. *American Journal of Sociology, 96,* 805–842.

Conger, R. D., Conger, K. J., Elder, G. H., Lorenz, F. O., Simons, R. L., & Whitbeck, L. B. (1992). A family process model of economic hardship and adjustment of early adolescent boys. *Child Development, 63,* 526–541.

Conger, R. D., Ge, X., Elder, G. J., Jr., Lorenz, F. O., & Simons, R. L. (1994). Economic stress, coercive family processes, and developmental problems of adolescents. *Child Development, 65*, 541–561.

Conger, R., Patterson, G. R., & Ge, X. (1995). It takes two to replicate: A mediational model for the impact of parents' stress on adolescent adjustment. *Child Development, 66*, 80–97.

Conger, R. D., Wallace, L. E., Sun, Y., Simons, R. L., McLoyd, V. C., & Brody, G. H. (2002). Economic pressure in African American families: A replication and extension of the family stress model. *Developmental Psychology, 38*(2), 179–193.

Cook, T. D., Church, M. B., Ajanaku, S., Shadish, W. R., Kim, J., & Cohen, R. (1996). The development of occupational aspirations and expectations among inner-city boys. *Child Development, 67*, 3368–3385.

Crocker, J., & Major, B. (1989). Social stigma and self-esteem: The self-protective properties of stigma. *Psychological Review, 96*, 608–630.

Currie, J., & Lin, W. (2007). Chipping away at health: More on the relationship between income and child health. *Health Affairs, 26*(2), 331–344.

Desai, S., Chase-Lansdale, P. L., & Michael, R. T. (1989). Mother or market? Effects of maternal employment on the intellectual ability of 4-year-old children. *Demography, 26*, 545–562.

Dressler, W. (1985). Extended family relationships, social support, and mental health in a southern black community. *Journal of Health and Social Behavior, 26*, 39–48.

Dubow, E. F., Edwards, S., & Ippolito, M. F. (1997). Life stressors, neighborhood disadvantages, and resources: A focus on inner-city children's adjustment. *Journal of Clinical Child Psychology, 26*, 130–144.

Duncan, G. J. (1991). The economic environment of childhood. In A. Huston (Ed.), *Children in poverty: Child development and public policy* (pp. 23–50). New York: Cambridge University Press.

Duncan, G. J., & Brooks-Gunn, J. (Eds.). (1997). *Consequences of growing up poor*. New York: Russell Sage Foundation.

Duncan, G. J., Huston, A. C., & Weisner, T. S. (2007). *Higher ground: New Hope for the working poor and their children*. New York: Russell Sage.

Duncan, G. J., Miller, C., Classens, A., Engel, M., Hill, H., & Lindsay, C. (2008). *New hope's eight-year impacts on employment and family income*. New York: Manpower Demonstration Research Corporation.

Edelman, P., Holzer, H. J., & Offner, P. (2006). *Reconnecting disadvantaged young men*. Washington, DC: Urban Institute Press.

Elder, G. (1974). *Children of the great depression*. Chicago: University of Chicago Press.

Elder, G., Nguyen, T., & Caspi, A. (1985). Linking family hardship to children's lives. *Child Development, 56*, 361–375.

Entwisle, D. R., Alexander, K. L., & Olson, L. S. (2000). Early work histories of urban youth. *American Sociological Review, 65*, 279–297.

Evans, G. W. (2004). The environment of childhood poverty. *American Psychologist, 59*(2), 77–92.

Evans, G. W., Kim, P., Ting, A. H., Tesher, H. B., & Shannas, D. (2007). Cumulative risk, maternal responsiveness, and allostatic load in young adolescents. *Developmental Psychology, 43*(2), 341–351.

Fishbein, D., Herman-Stahl, M., & Eldreth, D. (2006). Mediators of the stress-substance-use relationship in urban male adolescents. *Prevention Science, 7*(2), 113–126.

Flanagan, C. A. (1990). Families and schools in hard times. In V. C. McLoyd & C. A. Flanagan (Eds.), *New directions for child development, 46: Economic stress: Effects on family life and child development* (pp. 7–26). San Francisco: Jossey-Bass.

Furstenberg, F. F. (2000). The sociology of adolescence and youth in the 1990's: A critical commentary. *Journal of Marriage and Family, 62*, 896–910.

Garbarino, J. (1977). The price of privacy in the social dynamics of child abuse. *Child Welfare, 56*, 565–575.

Garbarino, J., & Sherman, D. (1980). High risk neighborhoods and high-risk families. The human ecology of child maltreatment. *Child Development, 51*, 188–198.

Gennetian, L. A., Duncan, G. J., Knox, V. W., Vargas, W. G., Clark-Kauffman, E., & London, A. S. (2004). How welfare and work policies for parents affect adolescents' school outcomes: A synthesis of evidence from experimental studies. *Journal of Research on Adolescence, 14*, 399–423.

Glasgow, D. (1981). *The black underclass: Poverty, unemployment and entrapment of Ghetto youth*. San Francisco: Jossey-Bass.

Goodman, E. (1999). The role of socioeconomic status gradients in explaining differences in US adolescents' health. *American Journal of Public Health, 89*(10), 1522–1528.

Goosby, B. J. (2007). Poverty duration, maternal psychological resources, and adolescent socioeconomic outcomes. *Journal of Family Issues, 28*, 1113–1134.

Gouldner, H. (1978). *Teachers' pets, troublemakers, and nobodies: Black children in elementary school*. Westport, CT: Greenwood.

Greenberg., M. (2007). Next steps for federal child care policy. *The Future of Children, 27*, 73–96.

Greenberg, M. H., Levin-Epstein, J., Hutson, R. Q., Ooms, T. J., Schumacher, R., Turetsky, V., et al. (2002). The 1996 welfare law: Key elements and reauthorization issues affecting children. *The Future of Children, 12*, 27–57.

Gutman, L. M., & Eccles, J. S. (1999). Financial strain, parenting behaviors, and adolescents' achievement: Testing model equivalence between African American and European American single- and two-parent families. *Child Development, 70*, 1464–1476.

Gutman, L., McLoyd, V. C., & Toyokawa, T. (2005). Financial strain, neighborhood stress, parenting behaviors, and adolescent functioning of urban African American boys and girls. *Journal of Research on Adolescence, 15*, 425–449.

H.R.1., 111th Congress, American Investment and Recovery Act. (2009). (enacted).

Hellenga, K., Aber, M., & Rhodes, J. (2002). African American adolescent mothers' vocational aspiration-expectation gap: Individual, social and environmental influences. *Psychology of Women Quarterly, 26*, 200–212.

Hill, M. S., & Sandford, J. R. (1995). Effects of childhood poverty on productivity later in life: Implications for public policy. *Children & Youth Services Review, 17*, 91–126.

Huston, A. C. (Ed.). (1991). *Children in poverty: Child development and public policy*. New York: Cambridge University Press.

Huston, A. C., Duncan, G. J., Granger, R., Bos, J., McLoyd, V. C., Mistry, R., et al. (2001). Work-based antipoverty programs for parents can enhance the school performance and social behavior of children. *Child Development, 72*(1), 318–336.

Huston, A. C., Duncan, G. J., McLoyd, V. C., Crosby, D. A., Ripke, M. N., Weisner, T. S., et al. (2005). Impacts on children of a policy to promote employment and reduce poverty for low-income parents: New Hope after 5 years. *Developmental Psychology, 41*, 902–918.

Huston, A. C., Gupta, A., Bentley, A., Dowsett, C., Ware, A., & Epps, S. (2008). *New hope's effects on social behavior, parenting, and activities at 8 years*. New York: Manpower Demonstration Research Corporation.

Huston, A. C., Gupta, A., Walker, J. T., Dowsett, C., Epps, S., & McLoyd, V. C. (2009). *The long-term effects on children and adolescents of a policy providing work supports for low-income parents*. Manuscript submitted for publication.

Huston, A. C., Miller, C., Richburg-Hayes, L., Duncan, G. J., Eldred, C. A., Weisner, T. S., et al. (2003). *New Hope for families and children: Five-year results of a program to reduce poverty and reform welfare*. New York: Manpower Demonstration Research Corporation.

Institute for Research on Poverty. (1976). *The rural income maintenance experiment*. Madison, WI: University of Wisconsin.

Jackson, A. P., Brooks-Gunn, J., Huang, C., & Glassman, M. (2000). Single mothers in low-wage jobs: Financial strain, parenting, and preschoolers' outcomes. *Child Development, 71*, 1409–1423.

Jarrett, R. L. (1995). Growing up poor: The family experiences of socially mobile youth in low-income African American neighborhoods. *Journal of Adolescent Research, 10*(1), 111–135.

Johnson, M. K. (2004). Further evidence on adolescent employment and substance use: Differences by race and ethnicity. *Journal of Health and Social Behavior, 45,* 187–197.

Kerpelman, J. L., & Mosher, L. S. (2004). Rural African American adolescents' future orientation: The importance of self-efficacy, control, responsibility, and identity development. *Identity: An International Journal of Theory and Research, 4,* 187–208.

Kershaw, D., & Fair, J. (1976). *The New Jersey income maintenance experiment.* New York: Academic Press.

Kim, I. J., Ge, X., Brody, G. H., Conger, R. D., Gibbons, F. X., & Simons, R. L. (2003). Parenting behaviors and the occurrence and co-occurrence of depressive symptoms and conduct problems among African American children. *Journal of Family Psychology, 17*(4), 571–583.

Kingsley, G. T., & Pettit, K. (2003). *Concentrated poverty: A change in course.* The Neighborhood Change in Urban America Series: Brief 2. Washington, DC: The Urban Institute.

Korenman, S., Miller, J. E., & Sjaastad, J. E. (1995). Long-term poverty and child development in the United States: Results from the NLSY. *Children & Youth Services Review, 17,* 127–151.

Kotchick, B. A., Dorsey, S., & Heller, L. (2005). Predictors of parenting among African American single mothers: Personal and contextual factors. *Journal of Marriage and the Family, 67,* 448–460.

Lamb, M. E. (1998). Non-parental child care: Context, quality, correlates, and consequences. In W. Damon (Series Ed.), I. Sigel, & K. A. Renninger (Eds.), *Handbook of child psychology: Vol 4. Child psychology in practice* (5th ed.). New York: Wiley.

Lareau, A. (2003). *Unequal childhoods: Class, race, and family life.* Berkeley, CA: University of California Press.

Larson, J. (1984). The effect of husband's unemployment on marital and family relations in blue-collar families. *Family Relations, 33,* 503–511.

Larson, R. W. (2000). Toward a psychology of positive youth development. *American Psychologist, 55*(1), 170–183.

Leventhal, T., & Brooks-Gunn, J. (2003). Moving to Opportunity: An experimental study of neighborhood effects on mental health. *American Journal of Public Health, 93*(9), 1576–1582.

Leventhal, T., Graber, J. A., & Brooks-Gunn, J. (2001). Adolescent transitions to young adulthood: Antecedents, correlates, and consequences of adolescent employment. *Journal of Research on Adolescence, 11,* 297–323.

Li, S. T., Nussbaum, K. M., & Richards, M. H. (2007). Risk and protective factors for urban African-American youth. *American Journal of Community Psychology, 39,* 21–35.

Light, A. L. (1995). *High school employment* (Discussion paper 95–27). Washington, DC: US Department of Labor.

Linver, M. R., Brooks-Gunn, J., & Kohen, D. E. (2002). Family process as pathways from income to young children's development. *Developmental Psychology, 38*(5), 719–734.

Loeb, S., Fuller, B., Kagan, S., & Carrol, B. (2004). Child care in poor communities: Early learning effects of type, quality, and stability. *Child Development, 75,* 47–65.

Luthar, S. S., Cicchetti, D., & Becker, B. (2000). The construct of resilience: A critical evaluation and guidelines for future work. *Child Development, 71,* 543–562.

Lynam, D. R., Caspi, A., Moffitt, T. E., Wikstrom, P., Loeber, R., & Novak, S. P. (2000). The interaction between impulsivity and neighborhood context on offending: The effects of impulsivity are stronger in poorer neighborhoods. *Journal of Abnormal Psychology, 109,* 563–574.

MacLeod, J. (1987). *Ain't no makin' it: Aspirations and attainment in a low-income neighborhood.* Boulder, CO: Westview Press.

Mahoney, J. L., & Bergman, L. B. (2002). Conceptual and methodological considerations in a developmental approach to the study of positive adaptation. *Applied Developmental Psychology, 23,* 195–217.

Mahoney, J. L., Larson, R. W., & Eccles, J. S. (Eds.). (2005). *Organized activities as contexts of development: Extracurricular activities, after-school and community programs.* Mahwah, NJ: Lawrence Erlbaum & Associates.

Makosky, V. P. (1982). Sources of stress: Events or conditions? In D. Belle (Ed.), *Lives in stress: Women and depression* (pp. 35–53). Beverly Hills, CA: Sage.

McLoyd, V. C. (1990). The impact of economic hardship on black families and children: Psychological distress, parenting, and socioemotional development. *Child Development, 61,* 311–346.

McLoyd, V. C. (1998). Socioeconomic disadvantage and child development. *American Psychologist, 53,* 185–204.

McLoyd, V. C., Jayaratne, T., Ceballo, R., & Borquez, J. (1994). Unemployment and work interruption among African American single mothers: Effects on parenting and adolescent socioemotional functioning. *Child Development, 65,* 562–589.

McLoyd, V. C., & Jozefowicz, D. (1996). Sizing up the future: Predictors of African American adolescent females' expectancies about their economic fortunes and family life course. In B. Leadbeater & N. Way (Eds.), *Creating identities, resisting stereotypes: Urban adolescent girls.* New York: University Press.

McLoyd, V. C., Kaplan, R., & Hardaway, C. (2010). Maternal psychological distress, child management, delinquent behavior and the moderating influence of neighborhood disadvantage in low-income families. Manuscript submitted for publication.

McLoyd, V. C., Kaplan, R., Purtell, K., Bagley, E., Hardaway, C., & Smalls, C. (2009). Poverty and socioeconomic disadvantage in adolescence. In R. M. Lerner & L. Steinberg (Eds.), *Handbook of adolescent psychology* (3rd ed., pp. 444–491). New York: Wiley.

Milne, A. M., Myers, D. E., Rosenthal, A. S., & Ginsburg, A. (1986). Single parents, working mothers, and the educational achievement of school children. *Sociology of Education, 59,* 125–139.

Mistry, R. S., Vandewater, E. A., Huston, A. C., & McLoyd, V. C. (2002). Economic well-being and children's social adjustment: The role of family process in an ethnicallydiverse low-income sample. *Child Development, 73,* 935–951.

Moore, K. A., & Driscoll, A. K. (1997). Low wage maternal employment and outcomes for children: A study. *The Future of Children, 7,* 122–127.

Morris, P. A., Huston, A. C., Duncan, G. J., Crosby, D. A., & Bos, J. M. (2001). *How welfare and work policies affect children: A synthesis of research.* New York: Manpower Demonstration Research Corporation.

Murray, B. (1996). Program helps kids map realistic goals. *American Psychological Association Monitor, 27,* 40.

Neblett, N. G., & Cortina, K. S. (2006). Adolescents' thoughts about parents' jobs and their importance for adolescents' future orientation. *Journal of Adolescence, 29,* 795–811.

Newman, K. S. (1999). *No shame in my game: The working poor in the inner city.* New York: Knopf and the Russell Sage Foundation.

NICHD Early Child Care Research Network (2000). The relation of child care to cognitive and language development. *Child Development, 71,* 960–980.

Orr, L., Feins, J., Jacob, R., Beecroft, E., Sanbonmatsu, L., Katz, L. F., et al. (2003, September). *Moving to opportunity for fair housing demonstration: Interim impacts evaluation.* Washington, DC: U.S. Department of Housing and Urban Development.

Parcel, T. L., & Menaghan, E. G. (1997). Effects of low-wage employment on family well-being. *The Future of Children, 7,* 116–121.

Phillips, D., & Bridgman, A. (1995). *Child care for low-income families: Summary of two workshops.* Washington, DC: National Academy Press.

Pogash, C. (2008, March 1). Poor students in high school suffer stigma from lunch aid. *New York Times,* p.1.

Posner, J. K., & Vandell, D. L. (1994). Low-income children's after-school care: Are there beneficial effects of after-school programs? *Child Development, 65,* 440–456.

Quane, J., & Rankin, B. (1998). Neighborhood poverty, family characteristics, and commitment to mainstream goals. *Journal of Family Issues, 19*, 769–794.

Quint, J. C., Bos, H., & Polit, D. F. (1997). *New chance: Final report on a comprehensive program for young mothers in poverty and their children.* New York: Manpower Demonstration Research Corporation.

Quinton, D., Pickles, A., Maughan, B., & Rutter, M. (1993). Partners, peers, and pathways: Assortative pairing and continuities and discontinuities in conduct disorder. *Developmental Psychology, 5*, 763–783.

Rankin, B. H., & Quane, J. M. (2002). Social contexts and urban adolescent outcomes: The interrelated effects of neighborhoods, families, and peers on African-American youth. *Social Problems, 49*, 79–100.

Roth, J. L., Murray, L., Brooks-Gunn, J., & Foster, W. (1999). Youth development programs. In D. J. Besharov (Ed.), *America's disconnected youth: Toward a preventive strategy* (pp. 267–294). Washington, DC: Child Welfare League of America.

Ruhm, C. J. (1997). Is high school employment consumption or investment? *Journal of Labor Economics, 15*, 735–776.

Salkind, N. J., & Haskins, R. (1982). Negative Income Tax: The impact on children from low-income families. *Journal of Family Issues, 3*, 165–180.

Sameroff, A., Gutman, L. M., & Peck, S. C. (2003). Adaptation among youth facing multiple risks: Prospective research findings. In S. S. Luthar (Ed.), *Resilience and vulnerability: Adaptation in the context of childhood adversities* (pp. 364–391). New York: Cambridge University Press.

Sanchez, B., Esparza, P., & Colon, Y. (2008). Natural mentoring under the microscope: An investigation of mentoring relationships and Latino adolescents' academic performance. *Journal of Community Psychology, 36*, 468–482.

Scarr, S. (1998). American child care today. *American Psychologist, 53*, 95–108.

Sears, H., & Galambos, N. (1993). The employed mother's well-being. In J. Frankel (Ed.), *The employed mother and the family context.* New York: Springer.

Shinn, M., & Gillespie, C. (1994). The roles of housing and poverty in the origins of homelessness. *American Behavioral Scientist, 37*, 505–521.

Sinha, R. (2001). How does stress increase risk of drug abuse and relapse? *Psychopharmacology, 158*, 343–359.

Smith, J., Brooks-Gunn, J., & Klebanov, P. (1997). Consequences of living in poverty for young children's cognitive and verbal ability and early school achievement. In G. Duncan & J. Brooks-Gunn (Eds.), *Consequences of growing up poor* (pp. 132–189). New York: Russell Sage Foundation.

Stanger, C., Dumenci, L., Kamon, J., & Burstein, M. (2004). Parenting and children's externalizing problems in substance-abusing families. *Journal of Clinical Child and Adolescent Psychology, 33*(3), 590–600.

Steinberg, L., & Silk, J.(2002). Parenting adolescents. In M. Bornstein (Ed.) *Handbook of parenting: Vol. 1. Children and parenting.* Mahwah, NJ: Erlbaum.

Strohschein, L. A. (2005). Household income histories and child mental health trajectories. *Journal of Health and Social Behavior, 46*(4), 359–375.

Task Force on Youth Development and Community Programs. (1992). *A matter of time: Risk and opportunity in non-school hours.* New York: Carnegie Corporation of New York.

Taylor, R. D., Casten, R., & Flickinger, S. (1993). The influence of kinship social support on the parenting experiences and psychosocial adjustment of African American adolescents. *Developmental Psychology, 29*, 382–388.

Taylor, R. D., Rodriguez, A. U., Seaton, E., & Dominguez, A. (2004). Association of financial resources with parenting and adolescent adjustment in African-American families. *Journal of Adolescent Research, 19*, 267–283.

U.S. Department of Health and Human Services. (2002). *Trends in the well-being of America's children and youth.* Washington, DC: Office of the Assistant Secretary for Planning and Evaluation.

Vandell, D. L., & Ramanan, J. (1992). Effects of early and recent maternal employment on children from low-income families. *Child Development, 63*, 938–949.

Wadsworth, M. E., Raviv, T., Compas, B. E., & Connor-Smith, J. K. (2005). Parent and adolescent responses to poverty-related stress: Tests of mediated and moderated coping models. *Journal of Child and Family Studies, 14*(2), 283–298.

Wandersman, A., & Nation, M. (1998). Urban neighborhoods and mental health: Psychological contributions to understanding toxicity, resilience, and interventions. *American Psychologist, 53*(6), 647–656.

Weisner, T. S., Bernheimer, L., Espinosa, V., Gibson, C., Howard, E., Magnuson, K., et al. (1999, April). *From the living rooms and daily routines of the economically poor: An ethnographic study of the New Hope effects on families and children.* Paper presented at the meeting of the Society for Research in Child Development, Albuquerque, NM.

Wilson, W. J. (1987). *The truly disadvantaged: The inner city, the underclass, and public policy.* Chicago: University of Chicago Press.

Wilson, W. J. (1996). *When work disappears: The world of the new urban poor.* New York: Knopf.

Wiltfang, G., & Scarbecz, M. (1990). Social class and adolescents' self-esteem. *Another look. Social Psychology Quarterly, 53*, 174–183.

Wyman, P. A., Cowen, E. L., Work, W. C., & Kerley, J. H. (1993). The role of children's future expectations in self-system functioning and adjustment to life stress: A prospective study of urban at-risk children. *Development and Psychopathology, 5*, 649–661.

Wyman, P. A., Cowen, E. L., Work, W. C., Raoof, B. A., Gribble, P. A., Parker, G. R., et al. (1992). Interviews with children who experienced major life stress: Family and child attributes that predict resilient outcomes. *Journal of the American Academy of Child and Adolescent Psychiatry, 31*, 904–910.

Yoshikawa, H., & Seidman, E. (2000). Competence among urban adolescents in poverty: Multiple forms, contexts, and developmental processes. In R. Montemayor, G. R. Adams, & T. P. Gullotta (Eds.), *Advances in adolescent development: Adolescent diversity in ethnic, economic, and cultural contexts* (Vol. 10, pp. 9–42). Thousand Oaks, CA: Sage Publications.

Zelkowitz, P. (1982). Parenting philosophies and practices. In D. Belle (Ed.), *Lives in stress: Women and depression* (pp. 154–162). Beverly Hills, CA: Sage.

Zimmer-Gembeck, M. J., & Mortimer, J. T. (2006). Adolescent work, vocational development, and education. *Review of Educational Research, 76*, 537–566.

McLoyd, V. C., Kaplan, R., & Purtell, K. (in press). Assessing the effects of a work-based antipoverty program for parents on youth's future orientation and employment experiences. *Child Development.*

School Racial/Ethnic Diversity and Disparities in Mental Health and Academic Outcomes

Sandra Graham

Contemporary health disparities research has at least three common themes. First, the focus tends to be on disparate health outcomes for different racial/ethnic groups, with people of color often faring more poorly than their White counterparts (see, for example, Sue & Dhindsa, 2006). Second, the concern has been with disparate outcomes associated with serious physical health conditions such as diabetes, obesity, cardiovascular disease, and HIV/AIDS, or serious mental illness such as depression or anxiety. Third, much of the discourse around these race-linked health disparities focuses on ways to alleviate disparities through, for example, access to quality health care and changes in life style.

In this article, I broaden the discourse by discussing health disparities in children and adolescents with an emphasis on the kinds of disparities that we see in schools—that is, children's social health once they walk through those school doors, their mental health, and their academic health. My focus is also on racial and ethnic disparities in these health outcomes, within the context of racial and ethnic diversity of classrooms and schools. Just as researchers who study serious physical and mental health disparities argue for structural and environmental changes to alleviate disparate outcomes by race/ethnicity, I am going to make a case for increasing school racial/ethnic diversity as a way to alleviate some of the social, emotional, and academic health outcome disparities that I discuss.

Why focus on school racial and ethnic diversity? Table 1 shows the changing racial/ethnic composition of K-12 public schools in the United States over the past 40 years, a change that has been fueled by the driving forces of immigration. The most striking pattern in Table 1 is the decreasing percentage of White students in the nation's public schools (from 80 to 57%) and the increasing percentage of Latino students (from 5 to 20%). The percentage of students who are African American remained about the same and the increase in the representation of Asian students has been slower, although in states of the Southwest such as California, Asians are the fastest growing racial/ethnic group. If these trends continue—and there is every reason to think that they will, given immigration that is primarily non-White and

S. Graham (✉)
Department of Education, University of California, Los Angeles, CA 90095-1521, USA
e-mail: shgraham@ucla.edu

G. Carlo et al. (eds.), *Health Disparities in Youth and Families*, Nebraska Symposium on Motivation 57, DOI 10.1007/978-1-4419-7092-3_4,
© Springer Science+Business Media, LLC 2011

Table 1 Changing Demographics of K-12 Population in the US

	Year		
	1968 (%)	1998 (%)	2008 (%)
White	80	67	57
African American	14	17	17
Latino	5	14	20
Asian/other	1	5	6

differential birth rates in these racial/ethnic groups—within a decade White students will no longer be the majority in our nation's schools, and public schools will be the first institution in this country without a majority of any one racial/ethnic group.

But at a time when the school-aged population is becoming increasingly ethnically diverse, are public schools also becoming more ethnically diverse? Walk through the doors of any randomly selected public school in this country. Sit in a classroom, eat in the lunchroom, stroll through the playground or hallways. It will be apparent that our schools are more racially segregated now than they have been in the past 40 years (Orfield & Lee, 2007). For example, the typical White student attends school where almost 80% of the students are White, and the typical African American or Latino student attends school where at least two-thirds of the students are from their racial/ethnic group. Moreover, the great majority of highly segregated ethnic minority schools are located in urban pockets of concentrated poverty, which puts their students at greater risk for poor academic outcomes.

To illustrate, Fig. 1 shows the racial/ethnic composition of the five largest central city school districts in the United States: New York, Los Angeles, Miami-Dade,

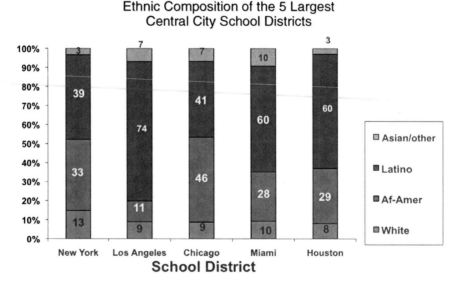

Fig. 1 Racial composotion of the five largest central city school districts in the United States. Source: National Center for Educational Statistics, Common Core of Data

Chicago, and Houston. In each of these school districts at least 85% of the students are nonwhite. If we were to examine the next five largest central city school districts (Philadelphia, Detroit, Dallas, San Diego, and Memphis), we would see similar patterns (NCES, 2007). I am not arguing that attending schools where there are no White children is intrinsically bad. Indeed, there is a growing constellation of *multiracial schools* that comprise three or more racial/ethnic groups other than White. The problem is that greater ethnic minority enrollment typically is associated with increasing poverty. Poor schools have fewer resources and more problems than wealthier schools and this is part of a whole syndrome of unequal opportunity and racial/ethnic disparities.

This is a critical time for studying issues about school diversity because the Supreme Court continues to roll back the progress made in the decades following *Brown v Board of Education* in 1954. Although psychological research played a pivotal role in the *Brown* decision, there has been relatively little systematic research on the psychosocial consequences of school ethnic diversity since the early studies in the 1960s and 1970s that followed *Brown*. That research, which yielded inconsistent and sometimes disappointing findings, all but disappeared by the mid 1980s (along with court-ordered desegregation), with little definitive evidence that attending a desegregated school either enhanced the self-views of ethnic minority youth or improved intergroup relations (see Schofield & Hausmann, 2004; Schofield, 1991). Ironically, one of the lasting legacies of the early research was that African American students reported higher self-esteem when they attended racially segregated rather than integrated schools, a finding that sheds little light on the psychological benefits of greater diversity (Gray-Little & Hafdahl, 2000). I think that the time is now right for developmental psychologists to re-kindle the spirit of *Brown* with new programs of research that examine how ethnic diversity in K-12 schools can promote healthy psychosocial development in children and adolescents and reduce some of the known racial/ethnic disparities in social and achievement outcomes.

In the remainder of this chapter, I describe a program of research that my colleagues and I have undertaken to study both the benefits and challenges of ethnic diversity in urban schools. I draw on my background as a developmental social psychologist with expertise on adolescence and on my theoretical grounding in social cognitive processes, such as the attributions that adolescents make about themselves and about other people. Using that framework, I have been conducting a longitudinal study of the social and academic adjustment of a large sample of youth from different racial/ethnic groups during the 3 years of middle school and across the transition to high school. First I review research from this longitudinal study on the experience of peer victimization in middle school to illustrate some of the psychosocial benefits of school ethnic diversity. Peer victimization is a good context for examining social and mental health disparities because it has well established linkages to these outcomes. Then I turn to some of the challenges of diversity as I describe our work on the psychosocial and academic adjustment of our participants following the transition to high school. School transitions are critical turning points that can sometimes be disruptive and therefore exacerbate pre-existing social and academic disparities among youth of different racial and ethnic groups. In keeping with the topic of this *Nebraska Symposium* volume, my goal is to demonstrate how a focus on school racial/ethnic diversity provides a context to stimulate new thinking about ways to alleviate racial and ethnic disparities in school outcomes.

I use the terms *race* and *ethnicity* throughout this chapter, so I want to be clear about how I define those terms. As in most social science research involving race and ethnicity, I rely on participant self-report to classify individuals into particular racial and ethnic groups. I am aware that the scientific basis for racial categories continues to be debated. Scientists from many disciplines agree that race is more socially constructed than biologically determined, in that the meaning of racial group membership changes across time and context, and the variability within racial groups far exceeds that between groups (e.g., Helms, Jernigan, & Mascher, 2005). I adhere to the American Psychological Association's social constructionist definition of race as "the category to which others assign individuals on the basis of physical characteristics, such as skin color or hair type, and the generalizations or stereotypes made as a result" (APA, 2003, p. 380). Thus I make no assumptions about the biological underpinnings of race or the immutability of racial classifications. I use the five racial categories in the US census (White, Black/African American, Asian, Native Hawaiian/Pacific Islander, and American Indian/Alaska Native) when referring to any of these specific groups. Ethnicity, in contrast, is defined as a social category that reflects a group's common history, nationality, geography, language, and culture (National Research Council, 2004). With common origins in Mexico, Latin America, or the Caribbean, Latinos/Hispanics can be of any racial group and the construct of ethnicity allows us to define their shared identity. I prefer the term *Latino* to *Hispanic* because it better captures that group's Latin American recent ancestry. I take the position that the terms *race* and *ethnicity* are distinct but not mutually exclusive and I often use them together in this article. However when referring to distinct research literatures (e.g., the racial achievement gap between Black and White students), I use the specific term most appropriate to that literature.

Psychosocial Benefits of School Racial/Ethnic Diversity: Peer Victimization in Middle School

What Is Peer Victimization?

Peer victimization—also commonly labeled *harassment* or *bullying*—is defined as physical, verbal, or psychological abuse of victims by perpetrators who intend to cause them harm (Olweus, 1994). The critical features that distinguish victimization from simple conflict between peers are the intention to cause harm and an imbalance of power between perpetrator and victim. Hitting, name calling, intimidating gestures, racial slurs, spreading of rumors, and social exclusion by powerful others are all examples of behaviors that constitute peer victimization. Note that my definition does not include the more lethal sorts of peer-directed hostilities such as those seen in the widely publicized school shootings. Although some of those shootings may have been precipitated by a history of peer abuse (e.g., Twenge,

2007), they remain rare events. My definition and focus here is on more typical and widespread types of peer harassment that affect the lives of many youth and that have been labeled a public health concern by the American Medical Association. Not only is peer victimization quite prevalent, it also is associated with a host of adjustment difficulties. Students who are chronic victims of school bullying often are rejected by their peers and they feel depressed, anxious, and lonely (Juvonen & Graham, 2001). Epidemiological studies of frequency and prevalence (e.g., Nansel et al., 2001) indicate that victimization peaks during the middle school years, at a time when the importance of peer approval to individual well-being is heightened (Simmons & Blyth, 1987). In light of these developmental patterns, early adolescents who are victims of peer harassment might be particularly vulnerable to adjustment difficulties.

We study peer victimization during middle school from a social cognitive (motivational) perspective. Figure 2 shows the conceptual model that guides our research. We believe that an individual's thoughts, perceptions, and interpretations of events are important determinants of subsequent behavior. We are particularly interested in how experiences with victimization relate to psychological adjustment (e.g., depression, loneliness, self-esteem) social adjustment, and academic adjustment. We are also interested in the kinds of attributions that youth make for being victimized and how particular attributions relate to specific adjustment outcomes. Attributions are answers to "why" questions: such as why did I get picked on? Or why doesn't anyone like me? (see Weiner, 1986).

Most importantly for this chapter, we examine how these social cognitive processes are shaped by the racial/ethnic context, which we operationalize as the ethnic composition of classrooms and schools. We do this in three stages. First we investigate the ethnic context as an antecedent to both peer victimization and to related adjustment outcomes (paths a and b in Fig. 2). Next we examine the ethnic

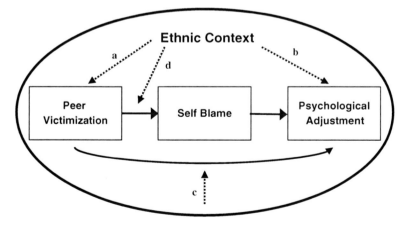

Fig. 2 Conceptual model of how the ethnic context influences relations between victimization, self blame, and adjustment

context as a moderator of the relationship of victimization to adjustment (path c). At the third stage we introduce attributions to explore how the ethnic context moderates the relations between victimization and self-blame (path d). The model underscores the importance of causal beliefs as a motivational framework and ethnicity as a central context variable for understanding the dynamics of peer victimization.

Ethnicity and the Antecedents of Peer Victimization

How might the ethnic context shape the experience of victimization (path a in Fig. 2) and feelings of vulnerability (path b)? Vulnerability was defined as feelings of loneliness, low self-worth, and perceptions of one's school as unsafe. We hypothesized that greater diversity would lessen experiences with victimization and feelings of vulnerability because in diverse settings students belong to one of many racial/ethnic groups who share a balance of power. We based this hypothesis on the definition of peer victimization as conflict that involves an imbalance of power between perpetrator and victim (Olweus, 1994). Mostly when we think about an imbalance of power, we think about size or age, as when bigger youth harass smaller peers, or when older students pick on younger targets. At the group level an imbalance of power can also exist when members of majority racial/ethnic groups (that is, more powerful in the numerical sense) harass members of minority ethnic groups (that is, less powerful in the numerical sense). When multiple ethnic groups are present and represented evenly, the balance of power is less likely to be tipped in favor of one ethnic group over another.

This hypothesis was tested in a large sample of about 2000 6th grade students who were recruited from 99 classrooms in 11 different middle schools in metropolitan Los Angles. The schools were carefully selected to yield an ethnically diverse sample, but within the constraints of a school district that is heavily Latino. Five schools were predominantly (more than 50%) Latino, three were predominantly African American, and three were ethnically diverse, with no single racial/ethnic group constituting more than a 50% majority. The ethnic breakdown of the sample was 45% Latino, 26% African American, 11% Asian, 9% White, and 9% multiethnic. In the Fall and Spring of 6th grade, students reported on experiences with victimization and feelings of vulnerability using well-validated rating scales (see Juvonen, Nishina, & Graham, 2006).

To measure ethnic diversity in the 99 classrooms and 11 middle schools that comprised our sample, we adapted a measure first used in the biology literature, called Simpson's index of diversity (Simpson, 1949). Scientists have used Simpson's index to capture biological diversity in terms of *richness* (the number of different species in a sample) and *evenness* (the relative abundance of those different species). Similarly, the concepts of richness and evenness can be employed to capture the racial/ethnic diversity of a school context—that is, both the number of different groups in the setting and the relative representation of each group.

The formula for measuring diversity (D_s) based on Simpson's index was as follows:

$$D_s = 1 - \sum_{1}^{g} p_i^2$$

where p is the proportion of students in the school who are in ethnic group i. This proportion is squared (p_i^2), summed across g groups, and then subtracted from 1. Substantively, this index calculates the probability that any two students randomly selected from a school will be from different ethnic groups. Values can range from 0 to ~1, where higher values indicate greater diversity (i.e., more ethnic groups that are relatively evenly represented, or a higher probability that two randomly selected students will be from different ethnic groups).

Figure 3 illustrates how ethnic diversity is calculated in three hypothetical classrooms that vary in diversity. The first pie graph depicts a classroom of Latino and African American students with low diversity: 85% of the students are Latino and 15% are African American ($D_s = 0.25$). The middle pie graph shows a classroom with the same two ethnic groups, but in this case they are equally represented. That classroom is more diverse by our definition ($D_s = 0.50$). Finally, the third pie graph captures the most diverse classroom ($D_s = 0.72$). It is comprised of four ethnic groups, all approximately equally represented. In our sample of 6th grade classrooms in 11 middle schools, classroom diversity ranged from 0 to 0.77 ($M = 0.48$, $SD = 0.22$) and school diversity ranged from 0.06 to 0.71 ($M = 0.48$, $SD = 0.19$), indicating substantial variation in diversity at both the classroom and school level. The correlation between classroom diversity and school diversity was 0.80 ($p < 0.001$), suggesting considerable overlap but not identical correspondence. There is no question in our mind that a great deal of de facto segregation occurs even in ethnically diverse schools.

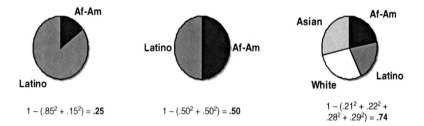

Fig. 3 Three examples of calculating Simpson's Diversity Index

Figure 4 shows how students' self-reported victimization and feelings of vulnerability in the spring of sixth grade varied as a function of classroom diversity (the data on school-level diversity were almost identical). Plotted here are the slopes predicting levels of vulnerability at high and low levels of classroom diversity. As diversity increased, self-reported victimization and loneliness decreased, whereas

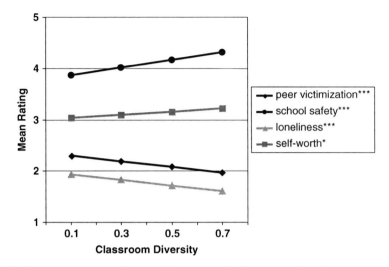

Fig. 4 Social vulnerability as a function of classroom ethnic diversity. (From Juvonen et al., 2006)

self-worth and perceived school safety increased. Thus our hypothesis was supported. When there was a shared balance of power, students felt less vulnerable at school. Although a few studies in the literature have examined peer victimization in different ethnic groups (e.g., Hanish & Guerra, 2000), to my knowledge this is the first study to document the buffering effects of greater ethnic diversity on the experience of victimization. Ethnically diverse schools can function as a mechanism for reducing racial and ethnic disparities by providing an opportunity for students to attend school where they feel safe and protected from harassment by numerically more powerful peers.

Ethnicity and the Consequences of Peer Victimization

In the next set of analyses, we examined how the ethnic context can influence the consequences of peer victimization (path c in Fig. 2). In Juvonen et al. (2006) we highlighted diverse schools to make the argument that as ethnic diversity increased, students felt less vulnerable. Here we focus on the consequences of victimization in the non-diverse schools for the same 6th grade sample. Non-diverse classrooms and schools—those with low scores on the Simpson Index—consist of both a majority ethnic group (Latino or African American in our sample) and one or more ethnic minority groups. Is one group more vulnerable to the consequences of peer victimization than the other? It seems reasonable to think that members of the numerical minority ethnic groups would be more vulnerable. That would be consistent with conventional wisdom, the way in which we think about an imbalance of power, and the reality that minority group victims may have fewer same-ethnicity friends to either ward off potential harassers or buffer the consequences of victimization.

On the other hand, consider what it must be like to be a victim *and* a member of a numerical majority group. Having a reputation as a victim when one's ethnic group holds the numerical balance of power might be especially debilitating because that person deviates from what is perceived as normative for his or her group. Social psychologists have used the term *social misfit* to describe the negative outcomes of individuals whose problem social behavior deviated from group norms (Wright, Giammarino, & Psrad, 1986). For example, in a study of boys living in cottages while attending summer camp, Wright et al. (1986) found that aggressive boys were most rejected when their cottage was low in perceived aggressiveness and withdrawn boys were most rejected when their cottage was low in behaviors associated with social withdrawal. The negative consequences of being a social misfit have been replicated in other social contexts such as laboratory play groups (Boivin, Dodge, & Coie, 1995) and naturalistic classrooms that could be characterized in terms of high and low levels of aggression and social withdrawal (Stormshak, Bierman, Bruschi, Dodge, & Coie, 1999).

With the sixth grade sample described above, we expanded the social misfit analysis by testing the hypothesis that the relations between victimization and maladjustment (i.e., loneliness and social anxiety) would be stronger for students who were both victims and members of the majority ethnic group (Bellmore, Witkow, Graham, & Juvonen, 2004). Peer nomination procedures were used to determine which students had reputations as victims. Participants were given a roster that contained the names of all the students in their homeroom, arranged alphabetically and by gender. Using that roster, participants were instructed to list the names of up to four students of either gender who fit each of three behavioral descriptions of victimization. Two of the victim descriptions portrayed physical and verbal harassment ("gets pushed around", "gets put down or made fun of by others"). A third description depicted indirect or relational victimization ("other kids spread nasty rumors about them"). The number of nominations that each student received for each item was summed and divided by the number of students in their classroom.

For each participant who had a score on the victim reputation measure, we created an individual level variable that we labeled *percent same ethnicity*. That variable described the proportion of peers in an individual's classroom who shared his or her ethnicity. The larger the proportion, the more likely an individual student is to be a member of the ethnic majority group. Thus the variable allowed us to examine the effects of being in a classroom with mostly same-ethnicity classmates (numerical majority status) in contrast to being a numerical minority. Hierarchical linear modeling was then used to examine the relations between victim reputation, numerical majority/minority status, and the outcomes of loneliness and social anxiety, while controlling for classroom level ethnic diversity (Simpson's Index) as a level 2 variable.

Controlling for classroom diversity in middle school, and independent of particular ethnic groups, the HLM analysis showed that victimization was related to more loneliness and social anxiety. More importantly for our purposes, that relationship was significantly moderated by ethnic majority-minority group status. Figure 5 shows the nature of that moderation for each adjustment outcome. Plotted here are

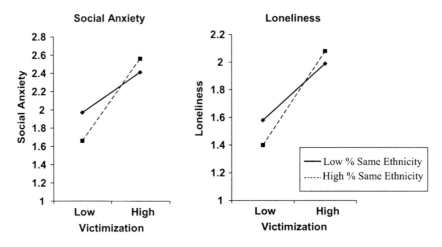

Fig. 5 Relations between victim reputation and adjustment for students residing in classrooms with a high versus low percentage of same ethnicity peers. (From Bellmore et al., 2004)

the regression slopes predicting loneliness and social anxiety at high and low levels of victim reputation (one standard deviation above and below the mean) for students who were high and low in the proportion of classmates who shared their ethnicity. Consistent with our predictions, the regression slopes describing the relations between victim reputation and both outcomes were steeper for 6th graders who shared their classroom with a larger percentage of same-ethnicity classmates (i.e., the numerical ethnic majority). In other words, and in agreement with a social misfit analysis, loneliness and social anxiety were greatest for victims who were members of the ethnic majority group.

These analyses lead me to my second conclusion about ethnic school diversity. It is not ethnic group membership per se but ethnicity within context that moderates the association between victimization and negative adjustment consequences. Being in the numerical ethnic majority group in contexts that are not diverse has its own unique risks that could be associated with disparities in psychosocial outcomes at school.

Ethnic Context and Attributional Mediators of Victimization-Adjustment Relations

Why is it that being a victim as well as a member of the ethnic majority group has negative adjustment consequences? That is, what processes might explain the relation between ethnicity in context and negative self-appraisals among victims? To address these questions, in the next study we turn to causal attributions as mediators of the relations between victimization and adjustment and the role of ethnic context (path d in Fig. 2).

When someone is a member of the majority ethnic group, repeated encounters with peer harassment, or even an isolated yet particularly painful experience, might lead that victim to ask, "Why *me*?" In the absence of disconfirming evidence, such an individual might come to blame themselves for their peer relationship problems, concluding, for example, that "I'm the kind of kid who deserves to be picked on". Self-blame and accompanying negative affect can then lead to many negative outcomes, including low self-esteem, and depression. In the adult literature on causal explanations for rape (another form of victimization), attributions that imply personal deservingness, labeled characterological self-blame, are especially detrimental (Janoff-Bulman, 1979). From an attributional perspective, characterological self-blame is internal and therefore reflects on the self; it is stable and therefore leads to an expectation that harassment will be chronic; and it is uncontrollable, suggesting an inability to prevent future harassment. Attributions for failure to internal, stable, and uncontrollable causes lead individuals to feel both hopeless and helpless (Weiner, 1986). Several researchers have documented that individuals who make characterological self-blaming attributions for negative outcomes cope more poorly, feel worse about themselves, and are more depressed than individuals who make attributions to their behavior (see Anderson, Miller, Riger, Dill, & Sedikides, 1994).

In earlier research we documented that victims of harassment were more likely than nonvictims to endorse characterological self-blame and they also felt more lonely and anxious at school (Graham & Juvonen, 1998). In the present 6th grade sample, we examined the mediating role of self-blame attributions and the possibility that relations between victim reputation, self-blame, and maladjustment would be moderated by classroom ethnic composition. We hypothesized that victims whose behavior deviated from local norms (i.e., victim status when one's group holds the numerical balance of power) would be particularly vulnerable to self-blaming attributions ("it must be *me*"). As the number of same ethnicity peers in one's social milieu increases, it becomes less plausible to make external attributions, such as to the prejudice of others, which can protect self-esteem and buffer mental health (Crocker & Major, 1989). Thus the temporal relations between victimization, self-blame and adjustment were expected to be strongest among ethnic majority group members. On the other hand, being a victim and a member of the minority group should facilitate external attributions to the prejudice of others ("it could be *them*"). For ethnic minority group members, we therefore expected weak relations between victim status, self-blaming tendencies, and adjustment. Finally, in ethnically diverse contexts, where no one group holds the numerical balance of power, we expected the most attributional ambiguity ("it might be *me*, but it could be *them*"). Here we thought there would be both indirect (mediated) and direct effects of victimization on maladjustment.

We used a combination of our classroom level diversity index and our individual level diversity (percent same ethnicity) to create three ethnic context groups: ethnic majority group students in relatively non-diverse classrooms, ethnic minority group students in relatively non-diverse classrooms, and students in ethnically diverse classrooms (see Graham, Bellmore, Nishina, & Juvonen, 2009 for details about how these groups were constructed). Victim reputation was measured as described above and the outcomes assessed were depression and low self-worth, again using well-validated indicators.

The instrument developed by Graham and Juvonen (1998) was used to assess self-blame attributions for hypothetical peer victimization. Participants were presented with the following scenario where they imagined that they were the target of peer harassment at school: "Imagine that you've just bought your lunch after waiting in line for a long time. As you are walking away, someone in the line sticks out their foot and trips you. You're not hurt, but most of your food spills on your clothes. The other kids in line start laughing at you."

Following the vignette, respondents rated on 7-point scales how much they agreed with 32 statements that captured what they might think and feel if the incident actually happened to them. The thoughts included six attributions designed to tap characterological self-blame (e.g., "This sort of thing is more likely to happen to me than to other kids", "Why do I always get into these situations?"). Note that we studied hypothetical or imagined experiences with peer victimization rather than actual experiences, which vary greatly between individuals and would be difficult to capture "in the heat of the moment". Some critics might view this as a methodological weakness. But as an attribution theorist, I believe that what individuals *say* they would think, feel, and do if certain conditions were present maps on to what they would *actually* think, feel, and do in those situations.

We gathered the victim reputation data in the Fall of 6th grade and the attribution and adjustment data in the Spring of the school year. The short-term longitudinal design accomplished two goals. First, it allowed us to make a stronger case for mediation. And second, it reflected our belief that the psychological consequences of having a reputation as a victim are likely to unfold over time.

Separately in each ethnic context group, structural equation modeling was performed to test relations between victimization, self-blame, and the maladjustment outcomes of depression and low self-esteem. Figure 6 displays the results of those analyses. For all three ethnic context groups, victim reputation was related to maladjustment and the endorsement of self-blame was linked to maladjustment; these

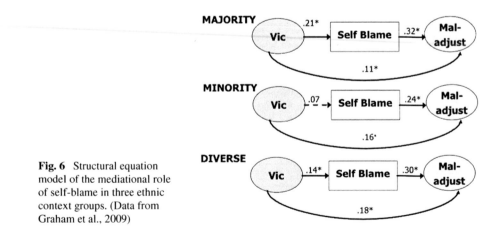

Fig. 6 Structural equation model of the mediational role of self-blame in three ethnic context groups. (Data from Graham et al., 2009)

findings are consistent with previous research. The critical path for our analysis was that between victim reputation in the Fall and characterological self-blame in the Spring. As predicted, the strongest evidence for the relation between victim status and self-blame was documented for students who were members of the majority ethnic group in their classroom, the weakest evidence was found for minority group members, while students who were in ethnically diverse classrooms were between these extremes. In other analyses involving comparisons of nested models, we found that the mediation model for majority group students was stronger than the one for students in diverse classrooms (Graham et al., 2009). Students who are both victims of harassment and members of the majority ethnic group in their classroom may be most vulnerable to attributions that implicate the self. These attributions, in turn, have motivational significance inasmuch as they partly explain the effect of victimization on maladjustment. This is one of few studies to test whether ethnicity as a context variable moderates a tested motivational sequence.

Summary

Let me summarize the studies that I have presented thus far. One of my goals in this chapter is to propose a framework for infusing ethnicity and ethnic context in the study of peer victimization. Within that framework, I have also attempted to make the case for studying the psychosocial benefits of racial/ethnic diversity in school. I believe that our research suggests three such benefits. In the first study on the antecedents of peer victimization (Juvonen et al., 2006), we showed that students felt safer, less victimized, and less vulnerable in ethnically diverse classrooms and schools. We hypothesize that greater ethnic diversity promotes a shared balance of power. When many ethnic groups are present and they are equally represented, the balance of power is less likely to be tipped in favor of one group over another.

In the second study on the consequences of victimization (Bellmore et al., 2004), we documented that being a victim when you are a member of the majority ethnic group can be especially painful because you deviate from what is perceived as normative for your group. We suggest that the emotional effects of perceived harassment are less painful in diverse as opposed to non-diverse settings because there are more reference groups, more social norms, and more opportunities for person-context fit.

In the third study on attributional mediators, we found that deviation from the norm can make someone particularly vulnerable to self-blaming attributions. We propose that greater ethnic diversity promotes more attributional ambiguity that can ward off self-blaming tendencies. Greater diversity among ethnic groups who share the balance of power discourages attributions for social failure to the self, while allowing for attributions to external factors or other causes that have fewer psychological costs. Attributional ambiguity has a somewhat different meaning in social psychology research on stigma, which highlights the threats to self-esteem when stigmatized individuals are unsure about whether to attribute negative outcomes to the prejudice of others or to their own personal shortcomings when, indeed, prejudice is the more appropriate attribution (e.g., Major, Quinton, & McCoy, 2002). But in social contexts where multiple cues are present and multiple causal appraisals of social predicaments are possible, attributional ambiguity can be adaptive if it allows the perceiver to draw from a larger repertoire of causal schemes.

Although I focus on attributional analyses, there surely are other factors that can explain the positive effects of classroom ethnic diversity. For example, perhaps teachers in more diverse classrooms do something different than teachers in non-diverse classrooms (e.g., addressing equity issues or promoting more cultural awareness). Or it could be that diversity fosters strong ethnic identity, which then acts as a buffer against general feelings of vulnerability. There are also challenges to school ethnic diversity, for in some contexts and for some outcomes, being a member of the ethnic majority group has self-protective functions. In the next part of this chapter, I turn to some of those challenges as I discuss findings from our longitudinal study when students transitioned from middle school to high school.

Psychosocial Challenges of School Racial/Ethnic Diversity: The Transition to High School

Ethnic Incongruence from Middle School to High School

The students whom we recruited from one of 11 middle schools and who remained in the longitudinal study transitioned to more than 50 high schools in the greater Los Angeles area. This transition sample allowed us to think about ethnic diversity in a more dynamic manner. We were particularly interested in whether changes in ethnic congruence—the extent to which an individual is racially or ethnically similar to other students in their school—affected the transition. For example, does it make a difference whether adolescents transition to high schools where there are many as compared to few members of their ethnic group, or whether the numerical representation of their ethnic group changes from middle school to high school? One might hypothesize that ethnic congruence—that is, similar numerical representation across transition settings—would be associated with better adjustment because there is less of a mismatch between the social context of the departing and receiving school (French, Seidman, Allen, & Aber, 2000). In a study of the transition to college that was consistent with this hypothesis, Adan and Felner (1995) reported that African American students who moved from high schools to colleges that were racially congruent experienced better school adjustment and received higher grades than their peers whose high schools and colleges were incongruent.

In the Spring of 8th grade and the Fall of 9th grade following the high school transition, we gathered data on students' feelings of belonging, academic worries, and school achievement as measured by grades and number of absences. We also calculated each student's percent same ethnicity in middle school and high school, reflecting the proportion of students in the school that matched the respondent's self-reported race/ethnicity.

Each participant's congruence change score was computed by subtracting the middle school percent same ethnicity (PSE) from the high school PSE (see French et al., 2000). Thus, for a student with a middle school PSE of 0.5 and a high school PSE of 0.25, the congruence change would be –0.25, indicating decreasing representation of one's ethnic group. We calculated these congruence change scores, standardized them, and then created an incongruent change group. That group was defined as students whose congruence change scores were 1 standard deviation below the mean, which meant that, on average, there were about 30% fewer of their own ethnic group in high school compared to middle school. We then examined how students' feelings of belonging, worries, and academic performance changed across the transition from 8th to 9th grade as a function of ethnic congruence or incongruence. These particular outcomes were selected to broaden our focus beyond peer victimization and to capture a set of psychosocial and adjustment outcomes that have been shown to be affected by the transition to high school (see Benner & Graham, 2009).

Figure 7 displays the findings for feelings of belonging, the psychosical variable that yielded the strongest effects of incongruence. African American (left panel) and Latino youth (right panel) in the incongruent group experienced decreases in feelings of belonging when they transitioned to a high school with significantly fewer members of their own ethnic group, whereas congruent students showed no change from Spring of 8th grade to Fall of 9th grade. The academic performance of incongruent students also was impacted, as measured by lower grades and a higher number of unexcused absences (see Benner & Graham, 2009).

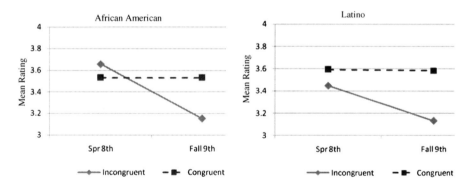

Fig. 7 Feelings of belonging from spring of 8th grade to fall of 9th grade for congruent and incongruent African American and Latino students. (From Benner & Graham, 2009)

These data call attention to an important issue in the study of school ethnic diversity and that issue has to do with the presence of a critical mass of same-ethnicity peers. In the legal discourse on diversity on college campuses, the notion of critical mass is discussed as "meaningful numbers" or "meaningful representation" of ethnic minorities to insure an ethnically diverse educational environment, while at the same time encouraging underrepresented students to participate in college life and not feel isolated or marginalized (*Grutter v Bollinger*, 2003). No ethnic group is likely to benefit from an ethnically diverse college campus or K-12 campus if their numbers are too small to combat feelings of isolation or marginalization.

What constitutes that critical mass? There has been very little empirical research on this topic, although speculations range in the 15–30% range. For example, it has been suggested that any ethnic group should be at least 15% of the school population to mitigate isolation and vulnerability to out-group hostility (National Research Council, 2007). Our findings suggest that it is not only absolute levels of ethnic group representation that need to be considered, but also *changes* in those levels across critical school transitions.

Worldviews and Racial/Ethnic Disparities in Achievement

We find it noteworthy that feelings of belonging, moreso than mental health outcomes such as loneliness and anxiety, were compromised across the high school transition for incongruent youth. Feelings of belonging capture social adaptation at school and establishment of positive social ties (finding one's niche, fitting in), a process that is more likely sensitive to changes in the critical mass of same-ethnicity peers in one's everyday ecology. Because the need to belong is a basic human motive (Baumeister & Leary, 1955; Leary & Cox, 2008), failure to satisfy that need can have serious adjustment consequences. For example, in the adult social psychological literature it has been documented that transitioning African American college students who questioned their belongingness on predominantly White college campuses were more likely to mistrust their educational institution, its teachers, and administrators (Mendoza-Denton, Downey, Purdie, Davis, & Pietrzak, 2002), to feel psychological distress, and to experience poor academic performance (Walton & Cohen, 2007).

When our sample transitioned to high school we began gathering data on a construct related to institutional mistrust as well as a set of inter-related constructs that together we labeled as school *worldviews*. Worldviews are an individual's core assumptions and beliefs about the way society and its institutions work (Koltko-Rivera, 2004). They encompass beliefs about what is and what ought to be, what is good and bad, and what relationships are desirable or undesirable. It does not matter whether these beliefs are proven or unproven. Whether accurate or not, a worldview is an interpretive lens that a person uses to understand his or her own reality. Some examples of worldviews studied in contemporary psychology are beliefs in a just world, or that people get what they deserve (Lerner, 1980); belief in human attributes as fixed versus malleable, as in entity versus incremental theories of intelligence (Dweck, 1999) and endorsement of the Protestant work ethic, or the belief that hard work pays off (e.g., Katz & Hass, 1988).

Our focus has been on worldviews regarding race and ethnicity in school contexts. Using well-validated instruments, ninth grade participants indicated their agreement with a set of questionnaire items designed to measure five constructs:

institutional mistrust ("When a teacher asks someone like me a question, it is usually to get information that they can use against us later") school interracial climate (e.g., "Teachers here like students of different ethnic groups to get along"), fairness of the school rules (e.g., "The punishment for breaking school rules is the same no matter who you are"); harshness of school discipline (e.g., "Students get in trouble even for breaking small rules"), and perceived discrimination at school (e.g., "Were you given a lower grade than you deserved because of your race/ethnicity?") (see Graham & Benner, 2010 for details). None of these variables in and of itself constitutes a worldview. But together I believe that they capture a set of interrelated beliefs about the legitimacy of school institutions and the way race and ethnicity function in those schools.

Person-centered approach. We used both person-centered and variable-centered approaches to analyzing the worldviews data. We started with a person-centered approach because we wanted to know whether there were differences among individuals or between groups of individuals in how the presumed indicators of worldviews related to one another. The person-centered approach can identify distinct categories of individuals in our sample who share similar patterns of worldviews. We used latent profile analysis to determine these categories.

The analysis suggested a 4-class model as shown in Fig. 8. The largest class (42%), labeled "positive worldviews" was comprised of adolescents who reported below-average levels of institutional mistrust, poor interracial climate, harsh school discipline, rule unfairness, and perceived discrimination. The smallest class (9%), labeled "negative world views," included adolescents who reported above-average

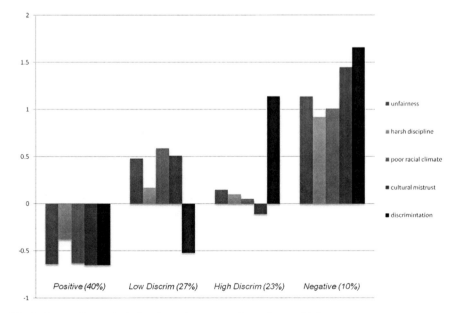

Fig. 8 Latent classes depicting the endorsement of negative worldviews

levels on all of the variables. We observed two other classes who differed primarily in terms of perceived discrimination, the one variable that directly tapped personal experiences. The larger of these two classes (27%), labeled "low discrimination" reported slightly elevated levels of mistrust, poor interracial climate, harsh discipline, and school unfairness, but below-average levels of discrimination. The other class (22%), labeled "high discrimination" was at the mean on all of the variables except perceived discrimination which was above average.

What individual and diversity-related school variables predicted membership in these classes? Here the findings were quite telling for the two extreme groups. Being male, African American, a low achiever, and transitioning to a more diverse high school with relatively fewer same ethnicity peers predicted membership in the negative worldviews class. In contrast, being female, White, and a high achiever who transitioned to a less diverse school with relatively more same-ethnicity peers was associated with the endorsement of more positive worldviews. Like feelings of belonging, positive worldviews about race and schooling can be compromised for some youth of color—African Americans in particular—when they attend diverse schools in which their ethnic group is a visible minority.

Variable-centered approach. Because worldviews can shape thoughts, feelings, and behavior (Koltko-Rivera, 2004), they have motivational significance. In the next set of analyses, we adopted a variable-centered approach to examine the relations between ethnicity, worldviews, and possible racial disparities in academic achievement. It has been well documented that African American and Latino youth do more poorly in school and on standardized tests than their White and Asian peers and that the achievement gap persists from childhood to adolescence (NCES, 2007). Here we reasoned that the endorsement of negative worldviews might, in part, explain some of these differences. African American and Latino students would be more likely to endorse negative worldviews than would White students and negative worldviews, in turn, would be related to (predictive of) academic performance documenting the achievement gap.

The analysis strategy proceeded in two steps. First we created a latent worldviews factor that was comprised of our five indicators: institutional mistrust, unfair rules, harsh discipline, poor racial climate, and experiences with discrimination. Confirmatory factor analysis showed that all of the indicators loaded on the latent variable. Next, we tested a meditational model using SEM in which the latent worldviews variable was hypothesized to mediate the relationship between ethnicity and academic achievement. To keep the analysis simple, we controlled for the effects of gender and school ethnic diversity. The results of the SEM, which yielded good model fit, are shown in Fig. 9.

Reading from left to right, the first set of paths shows the relationship between race/ethnicity and negative worldviews. With Whites as the reference group, these coefficients show that African American, Latino, and multiracial youth all endorsed more negative worldviews that did their White 9th grade classmates. Negative worldviews, in turn, were related to both lower overall grade point average at the end of 9th grade and increased absences. Grades capture adolescents' learning and academic skills, whereas absences are more a measure of behavioral engagement in

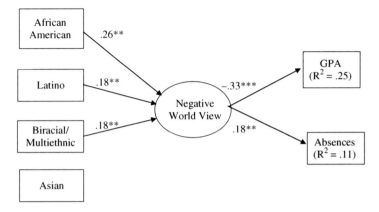

Fig. 9 Strutural equation model of the mediational role of negative worldviews in explaining the racial achievment gap

school (see Gutman, Sameroff, & Eccles, 2002). Thus we were able to document the effects of negative worldviews on both an ability-related and a behavioral measure of academic performance. More important for testing mediation, there were significant indirect effects from race differences to academic performance for all of these groups. That means that the academic performance differences between White students and their Black, Latino, and multi-racial peers respectively were partly determined by negative worldviews, with the strongest evidence of mediation for the Black-White achievement gap.

Further SEM analyses were carried out in which we included other possible psychological mediators of the achievement gap. These candidate mediators were a mental health latent variable comprised of depressive symptoms, loneliness, anxiety, and low self-esteem and a latent achievement attitudes measure that assessed respondents' and their close friends' endorsement of achievement-related activities (e.g., studying together, paying attention in class) (see Graham & Benner, 2010). We found that mental health and achievement attitudes were related to academic performance as we would expect: when students enjoyed better mental health and had positive attitudes about school work, they achieved higher grades and were absent less often. However, there were no racial/ethnic differences in these outcomes and no significant indirect effects. The indirect (mediated) effect of negative worldviews remained significant even after controlling for the influence of mental health and academic attitudes.

Much is written in the popular and scholarly literature about racial and ethnic disparities in achievement, and the search for explanations has continued relentlessly ever since reliable national data became available to the public. I would argue that we know a lot more about the structural variables, such as poverty and inadequate school resources, that perpetuate achievement disparities than we know about the psychological and cultural variables with explanatory potential.

A notable exception is research on stereotype threat, or the anxiety that can get activated when stigmatized students of color are confronted with highly evaluative achievement settings (e.g., Steele & Aronson, 1995). In one promising program of intervention research, African American middle school students were able to narrow the racial achievement gap when they participated in a self-affirmation task designed to reduce stereotype threat (Cohen, Garcia, Purdie-Vaughns, Apfel, & Brzustoski, 2009). However, the stereotype threat literature is not without its critics (e.g., Sackett, Hardison, & Cullen, 2004) and to my knowledge there are no studies that directly test the mediated effects of measured stereotype threat on the racial achievement gap.

Cultural explanations of the achievement gap have been similarly inconclusive (see Warikoo & Carter, 2009). Drawing largely on cultural-ecology theory (Ogbu, 1978), it has been argued that among so-called involuntary minority groups like African Americans, acceptance of mainstream values about working hard and school success may be perceived as threatening to one's social identity. Particularly during adolescence, African American youngsters may adopt oppositional identities whereby they show relative indifference, or even disdain toward achievement behaviors that are valued by the larger society. Fordham and Ogbu (1986) coined the term *acting white* to describe African American high school students' perceptions of their same race peers who work hard to do well in school. Most of the research in support of the phenomenon has been based on ethnographic studies that describe in vivid detail how high achieving Black youth sometimes conceal their accomplishments in order to avoid rejection and outright ridicule from same race peers However, the non-qualitative empirical literature in support of oppositional identity and its relation to the achievement gap is relatively weak. If there is pressure during adolescence to adopt anti-achievement attitudes as a means to gain acceptance by peers, this pressure appears to be equally evident among African American and White youth (e.g., Tyson, Darity, & Castellino, 2005).

Our findings on worldviews encourage me to think that studies of how students think about the relations between race/ethnicity and schooling—whether school administrators can be trusted and the degree to which students of all ethnicities are treated fairly—can shed new light on the psychological determinants of the achievement gap. This approach captures some of the dimensions of social psychological analyses of stereotype threat in that recognition of how others view one's racial/ethnic group are central. It also intersects with cultural analyses inasmuch as worldviews are a component of culture. I suspect that there may be more empirical payoff in studying worldviews as a cultural explanation of achievement disparities than oppositional attitudes and behavior.

Conclusions

The 50th Anniversary of *Brown v. Board of Education* in 2004 and the 2003 *Grutter v Bollinger* Supreme Court decision affirming ethnic diversity on college campuses as a "compelling government interest" refueled the public discourse on the benefits of ethnic diversity in K-12 schools. As I stated at the beginning of this chapter, American schools are drifting back toward the level of racial/ethnic segregation that precipitated *Brown* and there is little evidence that the public discourse has halted that drift. The June 2007 Supreme Court decision banning the use of race-conscious policies in the assignment of students to public schools in Louisville, Kentucky and Seattle, Washington (collectively known as the *Meredith* cases) was the most recent in a series of judicial rulings over the past two decades to successfully challenge the constitutionality of court-ordered school desegregation. Some of the most-cited research on the psychosocial benefits of ethnic diversity in K-12 schools has been portrayed as outdated, methodologically weak, too focused on Black-White comparisons, and theoretically impoverished—all of which can make it easier for critics of race-conscious policies to dismiss that evidence (National Research Council, 2007). As one critic so bluntly stated: "There are many things we need to do to address [the achievement gap], but worrying about the racial composition of schools is not one of them" (Armour, 2006, p. 27).

I believe that the best counterargument to such criticisms will be rigorous programs of research with theory-driven and testable hypothesis about *how* ethnic diversity reduces social, mental health, and academic disparities rather than *if* it does. Guided by research on peer victimization from a social cognitive perspective, I attempted to make the case for three benefits of racial/ethnic diversity during the middle school years. First, greater diversity lessens feelings of vulnerability because there is a numerical balance of power among different ethnic groups. Second, diversity fosters exposure to multiple norms, which then allows more possibilities for person-environment fit. And third, when interpreting the causes of victimization, greater diversity promotes more attributional ambiguity, which can ward off self-blaming tendencies. There are other testable hypotheses about how ethnic diversity promotes healthy development and reduces disparities between different racial/ethnic groups. For example, one might hypothesize that greater ethnic diversity facilitates the development of more cross-ethnic friendships over time and these friendships, in turn, foster better intergroup attitudes and relationship. Much has been written about contact between members of different ethnic groups and the power of cross-ethnic friendships to reduce prejudice, but these relations have rarely been tested either longitudinally or with child and adolescent samples (Pettigrew & Tropp, 2006). With an integrated focus on social, academic, and mental health, as well as intergroup relations, developmental psychologists will have the needed empirical base to make the argument that greater ethnic diversity in school can benefit all students.

I also argued that there are challenges to ethnic diversity that must be acknowledged and examined. Some of those challenges have to do with being a member of an historically marginalized racial minority group in a diverse setting, recognizing that minority status accompanied by coping with stereotypes and chronic experiences with race-based discrimination can take their toll and lead to negative worldviews, and understanding what constitutes a critical mass of same-ethnicity peers who can buffer the challenges of minority status. In addition, there are school structural factors, like academic tracking, that can limit the opportunity for cross-ethnic interaction even in the most diverse schools. In other words, there are complex issues about race, class, and schooling in contemporary America that are far beyond the range of our social cognitive perspective. What our perspective does offer, I believe, is a framework for asking some of the right questions in the continuing discourse on the value of school racial/ethnic diversity as a vehicle for reducing social, emotional and academic health disparities.

References

Adan, A., & Felner, R. (1995). Ecological congruence and adaptation of minority youth during the transition to college. *Journal of Community Psychology, 23*, 256–269.

American Psychological Association (2003). Guidelines on multicultural education, training, research, practice, and organizational change for psychologists. *American Psychologist, 58*, 377–402.

Anderson, C., Miller, R., Dill, J., & Sedikides, C. (1994). Behavioral and characterological attributional styles as predicotrs of depression and loneliness: Review, refinement, and test. *Journal of Personality and Social Psychology, 66*, 549–558.

Armour, D. (2006, November).The outcomes of school desegregation in public schools. Testimony prepared for the U.S. Commission on Civil Rights. *The benefits of racial and ethnic diversity in elementary and secondary education* (pp. 18–27). Washington, DC: U.S. Commission on Civil Rights, Briefing Report.

Baumeister, R., & Leary, M. (1995). The need to belong: Desire for interpersonal attachments as a fundamental human motivation. *Psychological Bulletin, 117*, 497–529.

Bellmore, A., Witkow, M., Graham, S., & Juvonen, J. (2004). Beyond the individual: The impact of ethnic diversity and behavioral norms on victims' adjustment. *Developmental Psychology, 40*, 1159–1172.

Benner, A., & Graham, S. (2009). The transition to high school as a developmental processs among multi-ethnic youth. *Child Development, 80*, 356–376.

Boivin, M., Dodge, K., & Coie, J. (1995). Individual-group behavioral similarity and peer status in experimental play groups of boys: The social misfit revisited. *Journal of Personality and Social Psychology, 69*, 269–279.

Cohen, G., Garcia, J., Purdie-Vaughns, V., Apfel, N., & Brzustoski, P. (2009). Recursive processes in self-affirmation: Intervening to close the achievement gap. *Science, 324*, 400–403.

Crocker, J., & Major, B. (1989). Social stigma and self-esteem: The self-protective properties of stigmas. *Psychological Review, 96*, 608–630.

Dweck, C. (1999). *Self-theories: Their role in motivation, personality, and development.* Philadelphia: Psychology Press.

Fordham, S., & Ogbu, J. (1986). Black students' school success: Coping with the "burden of 'acting White'". *Urban Review, 18*, 176–206.

French, S., Seidman, E., Allen, L., & Aber, L. (2000). Racial/ethnic identity, congruence with the social context, and the transition to high school. *Journal of Adolescent Research, 15*, 587–602.

Graham, S., Bellmore, A., Nishina, A., & Juvonen, J. (2009). "It must be *me*": Ethnic diversity and attributions for victimization in middle school. *Journal of Youth and Adolescence, 38*, 487–499.

Graham, S., & Benner, A. (2010). The motivational significance of negative world views about race and schooling. Manuscript under Review.

Graham, S., & Juvonen, J. (1998). Self-blame and peer victimization in middle school: An attributional analysis. *Developmental Psychology, 34*, 587–599.

Gray-Little, B., & Hafdahl, A. (2000). Factors influencing racial comparisons of self-esteem: A quantitative review. *Psychological Bulletin, 126*, 26–54.

Grutter v Bollinger, 539 U.S. 306 (2003).

Gutman, L. M., Sameroff, A. J., & Eccles, J. S. (2002). The academic achievement of African American students during early adolescence: An examination of multiple risk, promotive, and protective factors. *American Journal of Community Psychology*, *30*, 367–399.

Hanish, L., & Guerra, N. (2000). The roles of ethnicity and school context in predicting children's victimiztion by peers. *American Journal of Community Psychology*, *28*, 201–223.

Helms, J., Jernigan, M., & Mascher, J. (2005). The meaning of race in psychology and how to change it. *American Psychologist*, *60*, 27–36.

Janoff-Bulman., R. (1979). Characterological and behavioral self-blame: Inquiries into depression and rape. *Journal of Personality and Social Psychology*, *37*, 1798–1809.

Juvonen, J., & Graham, S. (Eds.). (2001). *Peer harassment in school*. New York: Guilford Press.

Juvonen, J., Nishina, A., & Graham, S. (2006). Ethnic diversity and perceptions of safety in rban middle schools. *Psychological Science*, *17*, 393–400.

Katz, I., & Haas, R. (1988). Racial ambivalence and American value conflict: Correlational and priming studies of dual cognitive structures. *Journal of Personality and Social Psychology*, *55*, 893–905.

Koltko-Rivera, M. (2004). The psychology of worldviews. *Review of General Psychology*, *8*, 3–58.

Leary, M., & Cox, C. (2008). Belongingness motivation: A mainspring of social action. In J. Shah & W. Gardner (Eds.), *Handbook of motivation science* (pp. 27–40). New York: Guilford Press.

Lerner, M. (1980). *The belief in a just world: A fundamental delusion*. New York: Plenum Press.

Major, B., Quinton, W., & McCoy, S. (2002). Antecedents and consequences of attributions to discrimination: Theoretical and empirical advances. In M. Zanna (Ed.), *Advances in experimental social psychology* (Vol. 34, pp. 252–330). New York: Academic Press.

Mendoza-Denton, R., Downey, G., Purdie, V., Davis, A., & Pietrzak, J. (2002). Sensitivity to status-based rejection: Implications for African American students' college experience. *Journal of Personality and Social Psychology*, *83*, 896–918.

Nansel, T., Overpeck, M., Pilla, R., Ruan, W., Simons-Morton, B., & Scheidt, P. (2001). Bullying behaviors among US youth: Prevalence and association with psychosocial adjustment. *The Journal of the American Medical Association*, *28*, 2094–2100.

National Center for Educational Statistics (2007). *Achievement gap: How black and white students perform on the national assessment of educational progress*. Washington, DC: Institute of Education Sciences.

National Research Council (2004). *Measuring racial discrimination*. Washington, DC: National Academies Press.

National Research Council (2007). *Race conscious policies for assigning students to schools: Social science research and the Supreme Court*. Washington, DC: National Academy Press.

Ogbu, J. (1978). *Minority education and caste: The American system in cross-cultural perspective*. New York: Academic Press.

Olweus, D. (1994). Bullying at school: Basic facts and effects of a school-based intervention program. *Journal of Child Psychology and Psychiatry and Allied Disciplines*, *35*, 1171–1190.

Orfield, G., & Lee, C. (2007). *Historic reversals, accelerating resegregation, and the need for new integration strategies*. Los Angeles: Civil Rights Project/Proyecto Derechos Civiles, UCLA.

Pettigrew, T., & Tropp, L. (2006). A meta-analytic test of intergroup contact theory. *Journal of Personality and Social Psychology*, *90*, 751–783.

Sackett, P., Hardison, C., & Cullen, M. (2004). On interpreting stereotype threat as accounting for African American white differences on cognitive tests. *American Psychologist*, *59*, 7–13.

Schofield, J. (1991). School desegregation and intergroup relations: A review of the literature. *Review of Research in Education*, *17*, 335–409.

Schofield, J., & Hausmann, L. (2004). School desegregation and social science research. *American Psychologist*, *59*, 538–546.

Simmons, R., & Blyth, D. (1987). *Moving into adolescence: The impact of pubertal change and school context*. Hawthorne, NY: Aldine de Gruyter.

Simpson, E. H. (1949, April 30). Measurement of diversity. *Nature*, *163*, p. 688.

Steele, C., & Aronson, J. (1995). Stereotype threat and the intellectual performance of African Americans. *Journal of Personality and Social Psychology, 69*, 797–811.

Stormshak, E., Bierman, K., Bruschi, C., Dodge, K., & Coie, J., & the Conduct Problems Prevention Research Group (1999). The relation between behavior problems and peer preference in different classroom contexts. *Child Development, 70*, 169–182.

Sue, S., & Dhindsa, M. (2006). Existence of disparities in health status and in receiving quality health care. *Health Education & Behavior, 33*, 459–469.

Twenge, J. (2007). The socially excluded self. In C. Sedikides & S. Spencer (Eds.), *The self: Frontiers of social psychology* (pp. 311–323). New York: Psychology Press.

Tyson, K., Darity, W., & Castellino, D. (2005). It's not "a black thing": Understanding the burden of acting white and other dilemmas of high achievement. *American Sociological Review, 70*, 582–605.

Walton, G., & Cohen, G. (2007). A question of belonging: Race, social fit, and achievement. *Journal of Personality and Social Psychology, 92*, 82–96.

Warikoo, N., & Carter, P. (2009). Cultural explanations for racial and ethnic stratification in academic achievement: A call for a new and impoirved theory. *Review of Educational Research, 79*, 366–394.

Weiner, B. (1986). *An attributional theory of motivation and emotion*. New York: Springer.

Wright, J., Giammarino, M., & Psrad, H. (1986). Social status in small groups: Individual-group similarity and the social "misfit". *Journal of Personality and Social Psychology, 50*, 523–536.

Social Identity, Motivation, and Well Being Among Adolescents from Asian and Latin American Backgrounds

Andrew J. Fuligni

Introduction

Youth from Asian and Latin American backgrounds, the fastest rising minority groups in American society, face numerous challenges to their successful development. The majority of these adolescents have immigrant parents and many of them were born in another country themselves, creating the need to adapt and adjust to a new and different society (Hernandez, 2004). The youths' families come from cultural backgrounds that include beliefs, values, and traditions that often differ from the dominant norms in American society. As ethnic minorities, they face social stereotypes that attempt to limit and constrain their abilities, resources, and potential (Fuligni, 2007). Large segments of these populations face significant levels of economic distress, with some Asian and Latin American groups evidencing the lowest levels of income, occupation, and education of all ethnic groups in the United States (Reeves & Bennett, 2003). Finally, adolescents from Asian and Latin American backgrounds consistently encounter substandard institutions and services, being more likely to attend low quality schools, live in high poverty and low resource neighborhoods, and have limited access to physical and mental health services (Fuligni & Hardway, 2004).

In addition to directly creating disparities in resources and opportunities, the challenges listed above converge to emphasize difference, exclusion, and a devaluing of adolescents' abilities and contributions to the larger society. Feeling as if one is being excluded and devalued is one of the most threatening social stressors, with significant implications for mental and physical health and one's ability to engage productively with institutions that are essential for societal integration (Dickerson & Kemeny, 2004; Eisenberger, Lieberman, & Williams, 2003; Fuligni,

A.J. Fuligni (✉)
University of California, Los Angeles, CA, USA
e-mail: afuligni@ucla.edu

G. Carlo et al. (eds.), *Health Disparities in Youth and Families*, Nebraska
Symposium on Motivation 57, DOI 10.1007/978-1-4419-7092-3_5,
© Springer Science+Business Media, LLC 2011

2007). Experiencing such devaluation during the teenage years is especially detrimental because adolescence is a critical period for the development of a sense of belonging, motivation, and purpose to make productive contributions. These psychological developments during adolescence, in turn, have consequences for more long-term mental and physical health, educational success, and occupational attainment during the transition to adulthood (Fuligni & Hardway, 2004).

Adolescents with Asian and Latin American backgrounds, therefore, must embark on these key development tasks in the face of significant barriers that exist by virtue of where they fall in the social and economic landscape of American society. The key question, then, is how do they do it? How do these adolescents develop a sense of belonging, motivation, and purpose when they consistently encounter both explicit and implicit messages that they are different, limited, devalued? In this chapter, I summarize a body of research that our research group has conducted over the past 10 years that suggests that in the face of their many challenges, Latin American and Asian youth obtain belonging, purpose, and motivation from their social identifications with their cultural and ethnic background and their families. Specifically, our work suggests that (1) cultural, ethnic, and family identities are heightened among these groups; (2) these social identities are predictive of a sense of purpose and motivation, and sometimes account for a greater sense of purpose and motivation among those from Latin American and Asian backgrounds than would have been predicted by the challenges that they face; (3) these social identities sometimes buffer adolescents from stress and other challenges; but that (4) cultural and family identities are not magic bullets—they can present challenges themselves and are limited in what they can do for adolescents in the face of limited opportunities and resources.

In the first section, cultural and family identities are defined and the theoretical basis for expecting them to play a role in the adjustment of youth from Latin American and Asian backgrounds is described. Next, the two major studies from which our findings are drawn are described, followed by a discussion of key results in regards to group differences in cultural and family identities as well as the implications of those identities for adolescents' adjustment and development. Finally, directions for future research and the implications of our findings for efforts to assist and improve the adjustment and development of these adolescents are briefly highlighted.

Cultural and Family Identity Defined

Our approach to cultural and family identity is consistent with the basic principals of Social Identity Theory (Tajfel & Turner, 2001). A social identity is the awareness that one is a member of a certain social category as well as the degree to which one places importance upon one's membership in that category. Literally thousands of experimental and naturalistic studies have examined the different dynamics of social identities, yielding a set of basic principles that hold up well across most identities and circumstances (Hogg, 2003). Three principles have been particularly relevant for our purposes as we have considered the role of cultural and family identities in the adaptation and adjustment of adolescents from ethnic minority and immigrant backgrounds. First, group identification is enhanced when functional use is made of group membership and when groups perceive external threat. That is, social identities become more salient when resources and opportunities are distributed according to group membership and when groups feel a sense of threat or challenge to their ability to access those resources and opportunities. Second, individuals with stronger group identification strive to be valued members of the group, are more likely to support the group, and to consider the group's goals and values when making important decisions. Finally, social identification can provide individuals with a sense of purpose, meaning, and motivation.

Cultural or ethnic identity has been commonly studied among ethnic minority adolescents and their families. Functional use is clearly made of ethnicity in the United States, with resources, opportunities, and numerous facets of daily experience being unequally distributed across ethnic and cultural groups. In addition, those from ethnic minority and immigrant groups are less likely to have equal access to resources and opportunities and are more likely to experience hostility and social threat, either explicitly or implicitly. As a result, ethnic minority and immigrant groups consistently have higher levels of identification with their ethnic and cultural background as compared to majority groups, such as those from European backgrounds (Phinney, 1990).

Family identity has been less commonly studied, but there is good reason to believe that family membership can act as a social identity for family members, above and beyond dyadic relationships within the family (Fuligni & Flook, 2005). Family identity represents the extent to which individuals believe they are part of a social group called the family and that membership in this group implies certain obligations and a desire to be a valued member of the group. There are a number of reasons why family membership can serve as a social identity. The family is the first and perhaps the primary social group to which children belong. Family membership is made socially obvious through salient cues such as physical appearance, surname, and shared residence. The family is a major source of opportunities and experiences for children, and family membership often entails shared beliefs and values that often differentiate families from one another. As a result, family membership is a significant way in which the social world is defined for children and adolescents, creating conditions that are favorable for the development of family as a social identity. Finally, given that ethnic group membership is largely defined by family of origin and that ethnic minority and immigrant families often perceive external threat, family identity is expected to be heightened among ethnic minority and immigrant groups. That is, even though traditions of familism and filial piety may exist in the cultural backgrounds of many ethnic minority groups, the simple fact of being an ethnic minority in the United States serves to maintain and even heighten a sense of family membership as a social identity (Fuligni & Flook, 2005).

Consistent with a social identity perspective, cultural, ethnic, and family identities should provide adolescents with a sense of belonging, purpose, and motivation.

In this sense, social identities can be a source of what has been called "eudaimonic well-being." As distinguished from hedonic well-being, eudaimonic well-being refers to a larger sense of purpose, direction, and meaning that one obtains in one's life (Ryan & Deci, 2001). It has been argued that developing this sense of connection, purpose, and direction is a key developmental task (Ryff, 1989, 1995). Eudaimonic well being can be stimulated by experiences of challenge and difficulty, which is why it has been suggested to be a particularly relevant aspect of adjustment and development among minority populations (Ryff, Keyes, & Hughes, 2003). Given the large body of work that has suggested that group identification can provide a sense of belonging and purpose, we believe that the cultural and family identities of adolescents from Asian and Latin American backgrounds that are made so salient by American society are important means by which teenagers from these families achieve these critical aspects of development. As described below, the findings from our studies suggest that this is indeed the case.

Study Descriptions

The findings presented in this chapter come from two longitudinal studies of adolescents from Latin American, Asian, and European backgrounds. The Bay Area Study of Youth from Immigrant families took place between 1992 and 2001 in a medium-sized school district in the San Francisco Bay area of California. The school district was selected on the basis of having sufficient numbers of students from Asian, Latin American, and European backgrounds and variation in immigrant status and socioeconomic background. Two cohorts of students, one in sixth grade and the other in eighth grade, were initially recruited from elementary and junior high schools in the district. Students completed self-report questionnaires during class time, and information on course enrollment, grades, and test scores was obtained from official school records. The students were followed at 2 year intervals, with additional new students recruited into the study at each successive wave, up to and including the twelfth grade, resulting in a total of approximately 1,000 participants during the high school years and representing more than 80% of the student population of the specific grade levels in the district. About 75% of the participants in the twelfth grade were interviewed by phone at one or both of two time points after high school: at 1 and 3 years beyond high school (younger cohort) or 3 and 5 years beyond high school (older cohort). Finally, at each of the post-high school waves, a subset of approximately 30 participants participated in qualitative personal interviews intended to provide a more in-depth view of the processes examined in the study. The Bay Area Study results that are presented in this chapter focus on the data collected during and after the high school years.

The second study was a longitudinal study of high school students in the Los Angeles area entitled the UCLA Study of Adolescents' Daily Lives. Approximately 750 students were recruited from three high schools in the Los Angeles metropolitan area on the basis on having sufficient numbers of students from Mexican, Chinese, and European backgrounds with generational and socioeconomic variability.

Starting in the ninth grade, about two-thirds of the enrolled students took part in the study by completing questionnaires during school hours. After completing the questionnaires, the students were given a packet of 14 daily diary checklists in which they were to check off the occurrence of a specified set of activities and experiences. The checklists were about 3 pages long and took 5–10 minutes to complete. Adolescents were told to complete each checklist before going to bed at night, place them in a sealed envelope, and were given a pre-programmed, electronic time-stamper that they used to stamp the envelope with the actual time and date of completion. Compliance was very high, with students completing well over 90% of the diary checklists. Students were followed every year of high school, with additional students recruited to the study at each grade level. Questionnaire and school record information was obtained each year, and the diary checklists were completed in the ninth, tenth, and twelfth grades. Finally, 16 students from the larger sample participated in an in-depth, qualitative interview each year.

Group Differences in Cultural and Family Identity

The social identity principles discussed earlier predict that cultural and family identity would be particularly strong among adolescents from Latin American and Asian backgrounds as compared to those from European backgrounds. Findings from our studies support this prediction and are described below, along with results that suggest the two social identities are closely linked to one another in adolescent development.

Ethnic labeling. In the Daily Lives study, we were interested in the types of ethnic labels that adolescents from Mexican, Chinese, and European backgrounds used to describe themselves (Fuligni, Witkow, & Garcia, 2005). Specifically, we wished to examine the extent to which adolescents used pan-ethnic labels (e.g., Latino or Asian) as compared to hyphenated labels (e.g., Mexican-American) or national origin labels (e.g., Mexican, Chinese). On the one hand, one might predict that the constant requirement to use pan-ethnic labels in completing official forms, applications, and standardized tests would lead adolescents to conform to the Americanized ethnic categorization system. Yet on the other hand, it is possible that the significance of cultural and ethnic identity for these teenagers may lead them to feel a stronger affinity to labels that at the very least incorporate their specific ethnic and cultural heritage, such as "Mexican" or "Chinese American."

Adolescents were presented with a list of ethnic labels that they could potentially use to describe themselves that included a mix of national origin, pan-ethnic, and hyphenated labels. Students initially were asked to indicate all of the labels that they used to describe themselves. Adolescents chose a mix of different labels, with those from Mexican and Chinese backgrounds selecting significantly more labels than those from European backgrounds. Those from Mexican and Chinese backgrounds were roughly equally likely to include hyphenated, national origin, and pan-ethnic labels in the collection of labels that they use to describe themselves, whereas those from European backgrounds were overwhelmingly most likely to use pan-ethnic

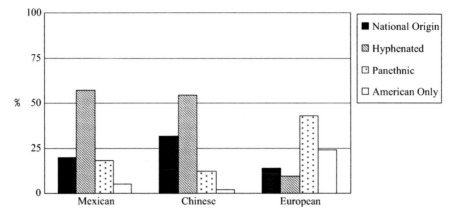

Fig. 1 Ethnic differences in adolescents' choices of the ethnic labels that describe them best. Adapted from Fuligni et al. (2005)

labels (e.g., White). These results suggest that during the years of adolescence, those from Mexican and Chinese backgrounds are exploring and trying on the different types of ethnic labels that are available to them in American society.

Yet when asked to select the single label that describes themselves most, adolescents from Mexican and Chinese backgrounds rarely chose pan-ethnic labels and leaned more toward hyphenated or national origin labels (see Fig. 1). Those from European backgrounds, in contrast, continued to use pan-ethnic labels. As predicted by a social identity perspective, therefore, adolescents from Mexican and Chinese backgrounds prefer to use labels that at least incorporate their specific ethnic or cultural heritage. In fact, many of these teenagers are attempting to combine that specific heritage with their sense of themselves as Americans. Although they rarely chose solely the "American" label to describe themselves, those from Mexican and Chinese backgrounds consider themselves to be a particular type of American with a specific type of ethnic and cultural background.

As one might predict, generational status differences do exist in Mexican and Chinese adolescents' choices of their ethnic labels. Foreign-born adolescents are significantly more likely to use national origin labels than hyphenated labels to describe themselves, whereas American-born adolescents prefer to use hyphenated labels (Fuligni et al., 2005). Birthplace, therefore, makes a difference in the ethnic categories with which adolescents' identify, and immigrant adolescents are less likely to feel that they can incorporate "American" into their ethnic labels. American-born adolescents, in turn, appear to believe that solely identifying themselves according to their parents' national origins is an option that is simply not available to them. Instead, they attempt to combine those origins with their identity as Americans. Interestingly, the generational status differences in adolescents' choice of ethnic labels remained consistent across the 4 years of high school. Despite the expectations that over time, adolescents from immigrant families would assimilate to the ethnic norms of American society, the foreign-born teenagers retain their identification with their national origins across a critical period of identity development and exploration (Fuligni, Kiang, Witkow, & Baldelomar, 2008).

Strength of cultural and ethnic identity. An additional aspect of cultural and ethnic identity is the extent to which adolescents from Latin American and Asian backgrounds identify with the labels that they use to describe themselves. We asked the participants in the Daily Lives study to complete commonly-used measures of ethnic identity, such as the Sellers measures of private regard and ethnic centrality (Sellers, Rowley, Chavous, Shelton, & Smith, 1997), in regards to the ethnic labels the participants indicated described them most. Private regard measured the extent to which students had positive feelings toward their ethnic group. Using a scale rang-ing from 1 (*strongly disagree*) to 5 (*strongly agree*), participants responded to eight items such as "I feel good about the people in my ethnic group," "I feel that the peo-ple in my ethnic group have made major accomplishments and advancements," and "I believe that I have many strengths because I am a member of my ethnic group." The centrality measure included seven items that assessed the extent to which the students' ethnic label was central to their definition of themselves. Using the same scale as described above, students responded to items such as "In general, being a member of my ethnic group is an important part of my self-image," "Being a part of my ethnic group is an important reflection of who I am," and "Overall, being a member of my ethnic group has very little to do with how I feel about myself" (scoring for this item reversed).

Consistent with a large body of research that notes higher ethnic identity among ethnic minority adolescents, those from Mexican and Chinese backgrounds reported significantly higher levels of private regard and centrality as compared to their peers from European backgrounds. Mexican adolescents were higher in private regard than Chinese adolescents, but the two groups were similar in their levels of cen-trality. These differences remained after controlling for parental education and did not vary across boys and girls. Interestingly, there were no generational status differences in the strength of adolescents' ethnic identification. That is, although adolescents from different generations used different ethnic labels to describe themselves, the strength of their identification with those categories were equally strong.

Similar results were obtained in other aspects of ethnic identity, including the extent to which adolescents spent time exploring their ethnic and cultural back-ground, and the ethnic differences in the strength of adolescents' ethnic identity remained constant across all 4 years of high school (Kiang, Witkow, Baldelomar, & Fuligni, 2010).

Family identity. Our examination of family identity among adolescents from Latin American and Asian backgrounds has focused on a specific aspect of their identification with their families that we have called family obligation. Consistent with the idea that social identification is closely tied to a desire to be considered a valued group member and a greater likelihood to support the group, family obliga-tion refers to a set of attitudes and behaviors that involve adolescents' willingness to support, assist, and respect the authority of the family. The tradition of children con-tributing to the family exists with the cultural background of many Latin American and Asian families (García Coll & Garrido, 2000). Given the links between family and cultural background, as well as the families' status as ethnic minorities in American society, we believed that family obligation would be particularly strong among adolescents from Latin American and Asian backgrounds.

Tenth and twelfth grade students in the Bay Area study completed a set of three measures designed to assess their attitudes toward supporting, assisting, and respecting the family (Fuligni, Tseng, & Lam, 1999). The first measure, current assistance, was designed to assess the students' attitudes toward engaging in household tasks and spending time with the family. Using a scale ranging from 1 (*almost never*) to 5 (*almost always*), adolescents indicated how often they thought they should engage in 11 activities such as "help take care of your brothers and sisters," "spend time with your family on weekends," "run errands that the family needs done," and "help out around the house." The second scale measured adolescents' beliefs about the importance of considering the needs, opinions, and wishes of the family, which was called respect for family. Using a scale ranging from 1 (*not important at all*) to 5 (*very important*), adolescents rated the importance of seven items, such as "make sacrifices for your family," "follow your parents' advice about choosing a job or major in college," "respect your older brothers and sisters," and "do well for the sake of your family." Finally, a third measure of future support assessed young adults' beliefs about their obligations to support and be near their families in the future. Using a scale ranging from 1 (*not important at all*) to 5 (*very important*), students indicated how important it was that they engage in six behaviors, such as "help your parents financially in the future," "spend time with your parents even after you no longer live with them," "help take care of your brothers and sisters in the future," and "live or go to college near your parents."

As shown in Fig. 2, all of the adolescents from Latin American (Mexican and Central/South American) and Asian (Filipino and East Asian) backgrounds reported a stronger sense of obligation to provide future support to their families as compared to those from European backgrounds. The same ethnic differences were observed for their respect for the family and their attitudes toward current assistance. These ethnic differences were large, sometimes reaching a full standard deviation in magnitude, and existed even after controlling for ethnic differences in socioeconomic

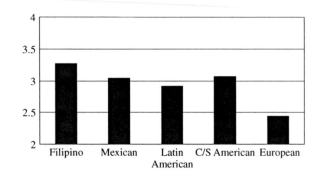

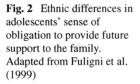

Fig. 2 Ethnic differences in adolescents' sense of obligation to provide future support to the family. Adapted from Fuligni et al. (1999)

status, family structure, and family size. Perhaps surprisingly, generational status differences in adolescents' sense of obligation to the family were small and inconsistent. The only notable pattern was that first generation (i.e., foreign-born) adolescents reported a stronger belief in the importance of providing support to their families in the future when they were adults, as compared to second and third generation (i.e., American-born) adolescents. Yet even with these generational differences, the third generation adolescents from Latin American and Asian backgrounds still had a stronger sense of obligation to the family than those from European backgrounds. The continuity of ethnic differences suggests that family membership, at least as represented by a sense of obligation to the family, is a significant social identity for those from Latin American and Asian backgrounds even after living for several generations in an American society that places great emphasis on independence and individuality.

Similar ethnic differences were observed in the Daily Lives study, with those from Mexican and Chinese backgrounds reporting a stronger sense of family obligation than their peers from European backgrounds across all three measures (Hardway & Fuligni, 2006). Interestingly, we have not observed ethnic differences in other aspects of family relationships, including emotional closeness or interpersonal conflict between adolescents and their mothers or fathers (Chung, Flook, & Fuligni, 2009; Fuligni, 1998). Adolescents from European backgrounds were similar to those from Mexican and Chinese backgrounds even in their reports of a generic sense of identification with their family (e.g., "My family is important to the way I think of myself as a person") (Hardway & Fuligni, 2006). Collectively, these findings suggest that adolescents from Latin American and Asian are not necessarily closer to their families in a general sense. Rather, they are different from those from European backgrounds in terms of this specific aspect of family identity that refers to a sense of obligation to support and respect the larger group.

Consistent with their attitudes, adolescents from Latin American and Asian backgrounds tend to provide more actual support and assistance to their families. Adolescents in the Daily Lives study reported the number of hours they spent each day helping the family in a variety of ways, including cooking, cleaning, sibling care, and helping parents with official business (Hardway & Fuligni, 2006). Mexican and Chinese adolescents spent significantly more time helping the family on a daily basis than those from European backgrounds. As shown in Fig. 3, these differences again were often quite large, with those from Mexican immigrant families spending twice the amount of time on family assistance as did those from families with European backgrounds. There was a slight, although non-significant tendency for students from Mexican immigrant families to also spend more time helping the family than those from non-immigrant families with Mexican backgrounds. Finally, variations in socioeconomic status did account for some of the ethnic differences in family assistance, particularly the higher levels of assistance among those from Chinese backgrounds as compared to those from European backgrounds. But the differences between those from Mexican and European backgrounds remained at least marginally significant after controlling for parental education and family size.

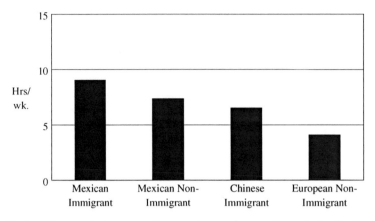

Fig. 3 Ethnic differences in hours spent per week providing assistance to the family. Adapted from Hardway and Fuligni (2006)

Family assistance continues into young adulthood, when it can take the form of living with the family or providing financial support to parents and siblings. Latin American and Filipino young adults in the Bay Area study were more likely than those from European backgrounds to both live with their parents and provide financial support to their families after high school (Fuligni & Pedersen, 2002). First generation young adults were more likely to provide financial support than their second and third generation counterparts. As with family assistance during high school, the financial support to families can be quite significant. Over 40% of those from Latin American backgrounds reported that they provided some financial support to their families as compared to only 16% of those from European backgrounds. Interestingly, the rates of family co-residence and financial support among those with East Asian backgrounds were significantly less than those from Latin American and Filipino backgrounds, in part because those from East Asian backgrounds were more likely to be attending 4-year, residential colleges at the time. As discussed later, a desire to do well in school and attend college is a correlate of a sense of family obligation, and qualitative interviews with some of the East Asian students suggested that their greater economic resources and high school achievement allowed them to fulfill their family obligation by applying to and enrolling in 4-year colleges and universities.

Ethnic and racial socialization. Important sources of adolescents' identification with their cultural background and families of origin are the messages that they receive about ethnicity, race, discrimination, and the importance of family from their parents. In order to assess their exposure to such messages, adolescents in the Daily Lives study were asked to complete the measure of ethnic and racial socialization developed by Hughes and colleagues (Hughes & Chen, 1997). Using a scale that ranged from 1 (*never*) to 5 (*six or more times*), participants reported how often their parents engaged in different activities that represented three aspects of ethnic socialization (Huynh & Fuligni, 2008). These aspects included cultural socialization

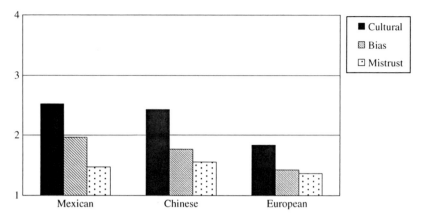

Fig. 4 Ethnic differences in adolescents' reports of ethnic and racial socialization from parents. Adapted from Huynh and Fuligni (2008)

(e.g., "In the past year, how many times have your parents encouraged you to read books concerning the history or traditions of your ethnicity?"), preparation for bias (e.g., "How many times have your parents told you that people might try to limit you because of your ethnicity?"), and the promotion of mistrust (e.g., "How many times have your parents done or said things to keep you from trusting students from other ethnic groups?").

As shown in Fig. 4, cultural socialization was more frequent than preparation for bias, which in turn occurred more often than the fairly rare promotion of mistrust. Adolescents from Mexican and Chinese backgrounds both reported significantly more frequent instances of cultural socialization and preparation for bias than did their peers from European backgrounds. Only those from Chinese backgrounds reported significantly more promotion of mistrust than their peers from European backgrounds. Interestingly, there were no generational status differences in any aspect of ethnic socialization. Finally, as might be expected, adolescents' reports of cultural socialization and preparation for bias were significantly related of students' sense of family obligation and ethnic identity across a variety of measures, with cultural socialization showing somewhat stronger associations ($rs = 0.25$–0.41) than preparation for bias ($rs = 0.10$–0.24). Reports of parents' promotion of mistrust, however, were generally unrelated to adolescents' ethnic identity and family obligation.

Linkages between cultural and family identity. It stands to reason that adolescents' cultural, ethnic, and family identities would be linked to one another. Theoretically, we have argued that the greater sense of family obligation among those from Latin American and Asian backgrounds is due in part to the fact that they are ethnic minorities in American society, having unequal access to resources and opportunities and experiencing various manifestations of social threat. Awareness of one's ethnic and cultural background and where one fits in the American social world, therefore, should be predictive of a greater sense of obligation to support and assist the family. As mentioned earlier, traditions of family support exist within the cultural background of many families with Latin American and Asian backgrounds. Finally, the parallel ethnic differences in ethnic and family identity discussed earlier suggest that the two would be related empirically.

Both our quantitative and qualitative findings suggest that this is indeed the case. Analyses of data from ninth grade of the Daily Lives study indicated that measures of ethnic identity designed by Phinney (Phinney & Rosenthal, 1992), which assessed adolescents' feelings of belonging to their ethnicity as well as their exploration of their ethnic background, were significantly and positively associated with the youths' sense of obligation to support and assist the family (Kiang & Fuligni, 2009). Adolescents who reported stronger feelings of ethnic belonging and a higher level of ethnic exploration also spent significantly more time helping their family on a daily basis. Cross-lagged correlational analyses suggested that ethnic identity at the ninth grade significantly predicted an increase in family obligation between the ninth and tenth grade, whereas the reverse direction of prediction was not significant. Finally, the higher levels of ethnic identity among those from Latin American and Asian backgrounds significantly mediated the stronger sense of obligation among these youth as compared to their peers from European backgrounds. Together, these results support the idea that ethnic and cultural identity is an important source of the family support and assistance among those from Asian and Latin American backgrounds, and partially explains why these adolescents place more importance upon family obligation than do those from the majority ethnic group. As a Chinese young adult in one of our studies concisely put it, "Asian families just have to, like, they have more at stake. They are just more familial orientated than, I don't know, American families in general" (Fuligni, Rivera, & Leininger, 2007).

Implications of Cultural and Family Identity

Adolescents from Latin American, Asian, and immigrant families clearly place a strong emphasis upon their ethnic and family identities. These identities stem in part from their cultural traditions and also result from their status as ethnic minorities in American society. A main focus of our research has been on the implications of these identities for adaptation and adjustment. As described below, ethnic and family identification are predictive of a sense of purpose and motivation and sometimes account for the greater levels of motivation seen among adolescents from Latin American and Asian backgrounds than would have been predicted by the many challenges that they face. These social identities sometimes buffer adolescents from stress and other challenges, but they can present challenges themselves and are limited in what they can do in the face of limited resources and opportunities.

Educational adjustment. The majority of our work on the implications of ethnic and family identity has been in the academic domain. In analyses of both the Bay Area and Daily Lives studies, we have observed that the strength of adolescents' ethnic identity and sense of family obligation consistently predicts academic motivation. Adolescents with higher levels of private ethnic regard and ethnic centrality reported a greater belief in the utility of education (e.g., "Doing well in school is the best way for me to succeed as an adult"), more interest in learning (e.g., "In general, I find working on schoolwork very interesting"), and greater identification with their school ("I feel like I am a part of my school"). These correlations tended to be somewhat small to moderate in magnitude (r range: 0.12–0.32), but were significant and consistent across ethnic groups (Fuligni et al., 2005). These findings are consistent with those from other studies in refuting the hypotheses of some observers that the ethnic identification among ethnic minority students would be an oppositional identity that refutes the value of schooling (e.g., Ogbu). The link with greater school identification is particularly interesting, in that it shows that greater ethnic identification actually may help Latin American and Asian students feel a greater sense of belonging to their schools.

Similar results have been obtained for family obligation. Adolescents with a stronger sense of obligation to support, assist, and respect the family also evidence higher levels of academic motivation (Fuligni, 2001; Fuligni & Tseng, 1999). Interestingly, although family obligation is associated with many different aspects of motivation, it appears to be most strongly linked to a belief in the importance and usefulness of education. Using high school data from the Bay Area study, we first removed the shared variance between adolescents' utility value of academics (e.g., "In the future, how useful do you think the things you have learned in math will be in your everyday life?") and their intrinsic interest in the subject matter (e.g., "In general, I find working on math very interesting"). Then, we examined the partial correlations of these two aspects of motivation with family obligation and found that the association with the utility value was significant but that the correlation with the intrinsic value was near zero and non-significant (Fuligni, 2001). These results suggest that family obligation seems to promote a belief in the value of the educational endeavor, but that it does not necessarily make students like school any more or less.

A significant finding in our work is that strength of ethnic identity and a sense of family obligation tend not to be associated with actual achievement in school. That is, the correlation between these identities and GPA tends to be non-significant (Fuligni et al., 1999, 2005). Similarly, ethnic identity and family obligation are not linked with a greater self-concept in one's academic ability, which is closely tied to actual achievement. Although a link between ethnic identity and achievement has been found in other studies, these results tend to be somewhat inconsistent, small in magnitude, and perhaps specific to African American students (e.g., Chavous et al., 2003). Our results suggest that ethnic and family identities are not magic bullets that will automatically promote higher performance in school. Academic achievement, as measured by course grades and standardized test scores, is multiply determined and strongly influenced by family resources, school quality, and other powerful structural factors. It should not be surprising that these social identities cannot outweigh the many challenges faced by many students from Latin American, Asian, and immigrant backgrounds.

Instead, ethnic identity and family obligation appear to help these students maintain a level of motivation and engagement with education that is greater than would be predicted by their socioeconomic backgrounds and actual achievement in school.

We have found that students from Latin American and Asian backgrounds report either similar or even higher levels of academic motivation across a variety of measures than do their peers from European backgrounds (Fuligni, 2001). We also have observed that adolescents from immigrant families evidence a greater belief in the importance and usefulness of education than do those from American-born families (Fuligni, 1997). In fact, the ethnic differences in academic motivation become even greater after controlling for students' actual achievement in school, suggesting that Latin American and Asian students have higher levels of motivation as compared to equally-achieving peers from European backgrounds. It is not that the motivation of these students is less effective, as demonstrated by the fact that the positive correlation between motivation and actual achievement is similarly strong across all ethnic groups. Rather, perhaps because of the many challenges that Latin American, Asian, and immigrant students face in their educational progress in American society, it simply takes more motivation to achieve the same level of academic success as their peers from European backgrounds.

Our analyses have shown that significant portions of this "extra" motivation to succeed in school on the part of adolescents from Latin American and Asian backgrounds is attributable to their higher levels of ethnic identity and family obligation. As shown in Fig. 5, the higher levels of motivation on the part of these students when compared to equally-achieving peers from European backgrounds become significantly reduced when controlling for adolescents' sense of obligation to the family (Fuligni, 2001). Similar results were obtained when controlling for the strength of the adolescents' ethnic identity and cultural socialization (Fuligni et al., 2005; Huynh & Fuligni, 2008). These findings are consistent with the idea that social identities help provide adolescents with a sense of purpose and motivation,

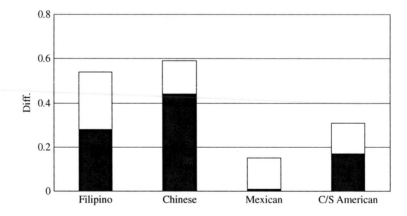

Fig. 5 Mediation by family obligation of ethnic differences in utility of education after controlling for grade point average (GPA). The total bars refer to the full differences as compared to students with European backgrounds with equal GPAs, and the clear portions refer to the proportion of the full differences accounted for by ethnic differences in family obligation. Adapted from Fuligni (1998)

which is a critical aspect of development during the teenage years. For those from Latin American and Asian backgrounds, identifying with their ethnic background and families helps them to be engaged in what can often be a very difficult road through the American educational system.

Family obligation is distinct from ethnic identity because in addition to being an aspect of social identity itself, it also implies the very real need to provide help and assistance to the family which actually could interfere with students' ability to succeed in education. Coupled with the sense of motivation to succeed in school that a sense of family obligation promotes, the demands of actually helping the family gives this aspect of family identity the quality of a double-edged sword for the educational adjustment of students from Latin American and Asian backgrounds. It appears that this sword cuts positively for most students, but it also can cut negatively for certain students under certain conditions. During the high school years, this may be particularly evident for adolescents whose family demands are high and frequent, such as the following student from a Mexican immigrant family who participated in our Daily Lives study:

> Sometimes I get irritated and frustrated about the fact that I have to sit late at night. Sometimes during the weekday, they [her parents] would go late at night to Wal-Mart or something, or to the market because they wouldn't have time during the day. So, she [her mother] leaves it up to me to watch my little brother or sister. Sometimes I have a lot of homework so I tell her I have homework and she says, 'Oh, you have to watch your brother and sisters.' I wind up staying up really late or sometimes I wind up finishing it in class.

The student effectively conveys the potential conflict between helping the family and studying for school that some Latin American, Asian, and immigrant students will experience when their parents work long hours and need assistance with the maintenance of the household. It is notable that despite this conflict, the student apparently gets her studying done by staying up late or doing it the next day in school. But one wonders if such a juggling act can compromise the quality of her studying and if it continues over time, whether it will begin to show up in diminished performance at school.

Findings from the Daily Lives study provide evidence that it is the consistency of the need to help the family on a daily basis that can interfere with achievement. Using the daily reports of family assistance across 3 years of high school (ninth, tenth, and twelfth grades), we examined the within-person associations between changes in family assistance and changes in grade point average (GPA) over time (Telzer & Fuligni, 2009b). Such within-person modeling allows us to essentially control for pre-existing individual differences that could confound such an association in traditional, between-person correlational and regression analyses. The results indicated that although that total time spent on family assistance was not associated with GPA, the total number of days spent helping the family was linked to significantly lower grades. That is, the GPAs of students from Asian and Latin American backgrounds were significantly lower in years that they spent a higher proportion of days helping the family. These results support the idea that helping the family is not necessarily problematic for academic achievement on its own. Rather, the inability of students and their families to compartmentalize those family demands to a limited number of days per week, thereby freeing other days for studying and doing homework, is what can take a toll on the students' achievement in school.

After high school, providing financial support to the family can get in the way of students' ability to pursue postsecondary education and fulfill their aspirations that were at least partially fueled by their sense of family obligation in the first place. Data from the Bay Area study suggest that youth who provide financial support to the family are less likely to enroll and complete 2-year or 4-year college programs (Fuligni & Witkow, 2004). Students from families who are experiencing financial distress seem to be particularly susceptible to this issue and it can occur at any time in their post-secondary career. This is exemplified by the following student from a Chinese immigrant family who graduated from a top 4-year university in part because of his desire to fulfill his parents' dreams and repay them for the sacrifices they made to come to the United States (Fuligni et al., 2007). Upon graduation, however, his father lost his job:

> I'm finding myself in a position where I have to possibly just start paying my parents' mortgage, because my father's laid off.... I mean I had all these plans to, like go to grad school and study graphic design like abroad. It puts a hamper on things...

In the subsequent conversation, this student talks about the feeling of "being torn" between pursuing advanced education and staying home to help the family. At the end of the interview, he suggests that he will pursue a compromise by which he will stay for a year to help the family before going off to graduate school.

Psychological well being. In our examinations of the implications of cultural and family identity for psychological well being, we have observed a pattern by which these identities tend to be more strongly associated with more positive well being as opposed to less negative well being. In the Daily Lives study, we analyzed the extent to which ethnic identity served to buffer adolescents from Chinese and Mexican backgrounds from stress on a daily basis (Kiang, Yip, Gonzales-Backen, Witkow, & Fuligni, 2006). Utilizing multi-level modeling, we examined whether the daily level association between stress and both positive (i.e., happiness) and negative (i.e., distress) well being varied according to adolescents' level of ethnic identity. As shown in Fig. 6, adolescents with low and moderate levels of private ethnic regard experienced lower levels of happiness on days in which they experienced more demands from family, peers, and school. Those with high levels of private regard, however, maintained a high level of happiness in face of stressful demands. Interestingly, the same moderation of daily stress was not observed for feelings of anxiety and distress. Adolescents with high levels of private regard were just as likely to report greater anxiety on days in which they experienced more stressful demands. Taken together, these results suggest that just as for educational adjustment, ethnic identity is not a magic bullet for mental health. Instead, it appears to help adolescents from Asian and Latin American backgrounds to maintain a level of positivity in the face of the stressful demands and distress of everyday life.

As with ethnic identity, we have found a sense of family obligation to be associated with more positive psychological well being. The young adults in the Bay Area

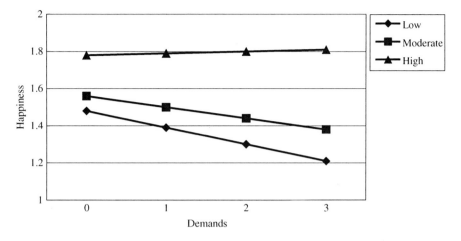

Fig. 6 Moderation of reactivity to daily stress by ethnic identity. Taken from Kiang et al. (2006)

study completed a measure of positive emotional well-being by using a scale that ranged from 1 (*none of the time*) to 5 (*all of the time*) to indicate how often they felt: "cheerful," "in good spirits," "extremely happy," "calm and peaceful," "satisfied," and "full of life" (Mroczek & Kolarz, 1998). Those with a stronger sense of obligation to support, assist, and respect the family reported significantly higher levels of positive emotional well-being, and this was true regardless of the adolescents' ethnic or generational background (Fuligni & Pedersen, 2002). In order to explore the possibility that very high levels of family obligation would be more negative than moderate levels, we also tested for the existence of curvilinear associations, but found none.

Although possessing a psychological sense of obligation to support the family may be conducive to positive psychological well-being, the actual need to assist the family on a daily basis may have different implications. Just as actually helping family had negative associations with educational performance despite the positive implications of a sense of obligation for motivation, demands from the family could potentially be too much for adolescents and create elevated levels of distress. We examined this possibility with extensive analyses of our daily diary data from the Daily Lives study (Telzer & Fuligni, 2009a). Each day, adolescents reported the amount of time they spent helping the family in a variety of ways, such as cleaning, cooking, and sibling care, and then whether they felt burdened by too many demands at home. Participants also reported their emotional states each day using subscales taken or adapted from the Profile of Mood States (Lorr & McNair, 1971). Adolescents used a scale that ranged from 1 (*not at all*) to 5 (*extremely*) to indicate the extent to which they felt distress (e.g., "sad," "hopeless," "nervous") and happiness (e.g., "joyful," "happy," "calm").

Employing multi-level modeling, we found that adolescents did indeed feel a greater sense of burden on days in which they spent more time helping the family. Yet adolescents did not report higher levels of psychological distress on days in which they spent more time helping the family. Instead, they actually reported slightly but significantly elevated levels of happiness when they provided more assistance to the family. These associations held up at the individual level, as well, indicating that adolescents who spent more time on average helping the family did not report greater emotional distress and instead reported elevated levels of happiness. There were no curvilinear associations between helping the family and psychological well-being at either the daily or individual level, and none of the associations differed according to adolescents' ethnicity, generation, gender, or socioeconomic status.

These results suggest that despite creating a sense of burden, providing assistance to the family elevates feelings of positivity among adolescents, including those from Asian, Latin American, and immigrant backgrounds. In order to test the possibility that this positivity resulted from the sense of meaning and purpose associated with the activity, we also asked adolescents to use a scale that ranged from 1 (*not at all*) to 7 (*extremely*) to indicate the extent to which they felt like a good son or daughter and a good brother or sister each day. As might be expected, adolescents' feelings of being a good family member were significantly higher on days in which they provided more assistance to the family. This sense of role fulfillment, in turn, mediated the previously reported association between family assistance and feelings of happiness. The same results were obtained at the individual level and again did not vary across ethnicity, generation, gender, and socioeconomic status. Together, these findings are strongly suggestive of the importance of family assistance for the psychological well-being of adolescents from Asian, Latin American, and immigrant backgrounds through the sense of meaning and purpose that it provides for them.

Physical health. Most recently, we have begun to explore the role that family obligation and assistance play in the physical health of adolescents. Approximately 70 students from Latin American and European backgrounds who participated in the Daily Lives study participated in a follow-up physical exam that took place an average of 8 months after they completed their diary checklists in the twelfth grade (Fuligni et al., 2009). As part of the physical exam, the participants' height and weight were measured for the computation of body mass index (BMI), an indicator of overweight status and obesity. In addition, intravenous blood samples were taken to allow for assays of indicators of systemic inflammation. One such indicator is c-reactive protein (CRP), a risk factor for the later development of cardiovascular disease (CVD) (Lagrand et al., 1999). An elevated level of CRP is considered to be a downstream indicator of chronic activation of the hypothalamic-pituitary-adrenal axis (HPA), which is one of the body's primary biological stress response systems. CRP has been shown to be associated with different types of stressful experiences and could be a primary pathway by which life stress can produce chronic health problems during adulthood. Given that Latinos increasingly appear to be at risk for several chronic health problems, including CVD, obesity, and type II diabetes mellitus, it is important to examine the potential sources of these problems earlier in development (Black, Ray, & Markides, 1999; Ranjit et al., 2007).

Results indicated that adolescents who spent more time helping the family on a daily basis during the twelfth grade showed elevated levels of CRP many months afterward, even after accounting for the higher BMI of these youth. Although relatively few teenagers had amounts of CRP that entered the "high risk" category, one does not expect to find particularly high CRP amounts at such a young age. These results suggest that although spending more time helping the family does not create feelings of psychological stress, high levels of family assistance may take a physical toll that the adolescent cannot appraise psychologically. In some ways, this can be seen as similar to the toll that high levels of actual family assistance can play on students' educational adjustment that was reported earlier. As a critical social identity in the lives of adolescents from Asian and Latin American backgrounds, family obligation can provide both benefits and challenges to the development of these youth.

Nevertheless, the important role played by the sense of meaning and purpose that family assistance provides to adolescents was evident even in these biological measures of health. Individual differences in the daily association between family assistance and role fulfillment (i.e., feeling like a good child or sibling) were obtained from multi-level models. That is, although most adolescents on average felt more like a good family member on days in which they helped the family, this association was stronger for some adolescents more than others, which we interpreted as an indicator of adolescents who obtained more role fulfillment from helping the family. We then examined whether the daily association between family assistance and role fulfillment varied according to levels of CRP (see Fig. 7). Adolescents with levels of CRP that were at one standard deviation below the mean showed a significantly stronger daily association as compared to those with levels of CRP at the mean or one standard deviation above the mean. Those who obtained more role fulfillment from helping the family, therefore, had the lowest levels of CRP. These results point to the need to discover why some adolescents obtain more role fulfillment from family assistance than others, but they also highlight the significance of

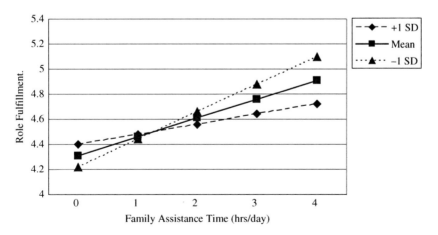

Fig. 7 Daily association between family assistance and role fulfillment according to levels of CRP. Taken from Fuligni et al. (2009)

the sense of meaning and purpose adolescents derive from their social identities for the development and adjustment of youth from ethnically diverse backgrounds.

Conclusion

Cultural and family identities are strong and remain strong across generations of adolescents from Asian and Latin American backgrounds in American society. These two linked social identities, in turn, enable teenagers to maintain a sense of purpose, meaning, and motivation in the face of the many social and economic challenges that they face as ethnic minorities and immigrants in American society. Specifically, the correlates of cultural and family identity—higher academic motivation, more emotional positivity, and a greater sense of role fulfillment—reflect what has been referred to as eudaimonic well-being, a key aspect of development that is especially relevant for ethnic and racial minorities who experience social threat and exclusion (Ryff et al., 2003). For adolescents from these backgrounds, cultural and family identities play important roles in the development of eudaimonic well-being at a critical time of identity development when minority adolescents confront both implicit and explicit messages that they are different, excluded, and devalued.

Yet it should be emphasized that cultural and family identities are not a panacea, and that they are no replacement for the provision of resources, information, and opportunities that are critical to educational attainment and the avoidance of mental distress and physical illness. We have had no evidence in our studies that either cultural or family identities are predictive of higher academic achievement, lower psychological distress, or better physical health by themselves. In fact, these identities sometimes present additional challenges themselves, as evidenced by associations between actual family assistance and lowered educational achievement and heightened inflammatory processes.

The critical role of access to resources, information, and opportunities is evident in the dramatic differences in educational and physical health outcomes between these two ethnic groups. Despite reporting relatively equal levels of cultural and family identity, adolescents from Asian backgrounds in the United States consistently achieve higher levels of academic success and educational attainment, and are significantly lower in many health risk factors than those from Latin American backgrounds (Fuligni & Hardway, 2004). These differences are due, in large part, to several advantages among those from Asian backgrounds in terms of economic resources and social opportunities as compared to those from Latin American backgrounds. Asian parents have higher levels of education, occupation, and income than Latin American parents. Asian adolescents also are more likely to attend better schools with greater resources, and sometimes are advantaged in terms of the expectations teachers and school personnel have for their potential. Finally, the greater proportion of more highly educated families in the Asian community results in a more effective social network by which critical information about educational opportunities, requirements, and pathways can be obtained by less educated members of the same community (Zhou, Lee, Vallejo, Tofoya-Estrada, & Xiong,

2008). It is not that adolescents from Asian families are advantaged, per se, as they often experience more social and economic challenges than their counterparts from European backgrounds. But the combination of strong cultural and family identities with the better resources that they can access leads them to have better educational and health outcomes than their peers from Latin American backgrounds.

Programs and policies that emphasize only cultural and social identity, therefore, are unlikely to gain much ground in minimizing the disparities that are evident in many developmental outcomes. But intervention efforts that include attention to these identities at the same time as providing needed resources, information, and opportunities should have a strong chance of succeeding because they provide the tools for success while at the same time helping adolescents from Latin American and Asian backgrounds to maintain a sense of purpose, meaning, and motivation as they attempt to accomplish their goals. One such program is the Puente Project, which focuses on providing Latino high school students in California with the informational and social resources necessary in order to be eligible for college enrollment while also supporting their cultural and family traditions (American Youth Policy Forum, 2001). Another includes the Bridges to High School program developed by Gonzales and colleagues as a way to incorporate cultural and family values into a psychological and academic intervention program (Gonzales, Dumka, Mauricio, & Germán, 2007). In a sense, what is recommended is a classic integration of the old and the new: help teenagers from Latin American and Asian backgrounds maintain their sense of themselves culturally and as valued members of their family, while simultaneously providing them with equal access to the skills and resources necessary for healthy development in American society.

References

American Youth Policy Forum (2001). *Raising minority achievement*. Washington, DC: American Youth Policy Forum.

Black, S. A., Ray, L. A., & Markides, K. S. (1999). The prevalence and health burden of self reported diabetes in older Mexican Americans: Findings from the Hispanic Established Populations for Epidemiologic Studies of the Elderly. *American Journal of Public Health, 89*, 546–552.

Chavous, T. M., Bernat, D. H., Schmeelk-Cone, K., Caldwell, C. H., Kohn-Wood, L., & Zimmerman, M. A. (2003). Racial identity and academic attainment among African American adolescents. *Child Development, 74*(4), 1076–1090.

Chung, G., Flook, L., & Fuligni, A. J. (2009). Daily family conflict among adolescents from Latin American, Asian, and European backgrounds. *Developmental Psychology, 45*, 1406–1416.

Dickerson, S. S., & Kemeny, M. E. (2004). Acute stressors and cortisol responses: A theoretical integration and synthesis of laboratory research. *Psychological Bulletin, 130*(3), 355–391.

Eisenberger, N. I., Lieberman, M. D., & Williams, K. D. (2003). Does rejection hurt? An fMRI study of social exclusion. *Science, 302*, 290–292.

Fuligni, A. J. (1997). The academic achievement of adolescents from immigrant families: The roles of family background, attitudes, and behavior. *Child Development, 68*(2), 351–363.

Fuligni, A. J. (1998). Parental authority, adolescent autonomy, and parent-adolescent relationships: A study of adolescents from Mexican, Chinese, Filipino, and European backgrounds. *Developmental Psychology, 34*, 782–792.

Fuligni, A. J. (2001). Family obligation and the academic motivation of adolescents from Asian, Latin American, and European backgrounds. In A. Fuligni (Ed.), *Family obligation and assistance during adolescence: Contextual variations and developmental implications, (New Directions in Child and Adolescent Development Monograph)* (pp. 61–76). San Francisco: Jossey-Bass.

Fuligni, A. J. (Ed.). (2007). *Contesting stereoypes, creating identities: Social categories, social identities, and educational participation.* New York: Russell Sage Foundation Press.

Fuligni, A. J., & Flook, L. (2005). A social identity approach to ethnic differences in family relationships during adolescence. In R. Kail (Ed.), *Advances in child development and behavior.* New York: Academic Press.

Fuligni, A. J., & Hardway, C. (2004). Preparing diverse adolescents for the transition to adulthood. *The Future of Children, 14*(2), 99–119.

Fuligni, A. J., Kiang, L., Witkow, M. R., & Baldelomar, O. (2008). Stability and change in ethnic labeling among adolescents from Asian and Latin American immigrant families. *Child Development, 79*(4), 944–956.

Fuligni, A. J., & Pedersen, S. (2002). Family obligation and the transition to young adulthood. *Developmental Psychology, 38*(5), 856–868.

Fuligni, A. J., Rivera, G. J., & Leininger, A. (2007). Family identity and the educational progress of adolescents from Asian and Latin American backgrounds. In A. J. Fuligni (Ed.), *Contesting stereotypes and creating identities: Social categories, social identities, and educational participation* (pp. 239–264). New York: Russell Sage Foundation Press.

Fuligni, A. J., Telzer, E. H., Bower, J., Irwin, M. R., Kiang, L., & Cole, S. R. (2009). Daily family assistance and inflammation among adolescents from Latin American and European backgrounds. *Brian, Behavior, and Immunity, 23*, 803–809.

Fuligni, A. J., & Tseng, V. (1999). Family obligations and the achievement motivation of children from immigrant and American-born families. In T. Urdan (Ed.), *Advances in motivation and achievement* (pp. 159–184). Stamford, CT: JAI Press, Inc.

Fuligni, A. J., Tseng, V., & Lam, M. (1999). Attitudes toward family obligations among American adolescents from Asian, Latin American, and European backgrounds. *Child Development, 70*(4), 1030–1040.

Fuligni, A. J., & Witkow, M. (2004). The postsecondary educational progress of youth from immigrant families. *Journal of Research on Adolescence, 14*(2), 159–183.

Fuligni, A. J., Witkow, M., & Garcia, C. (2005). Ethnic identity and the academic adjustment of adolescents from Mexican, Chinese, and European backgrounds. *Developmental Psychology, 41*(5), 799–811.

García Coll, C., & Garrido, M. (2000). Minorities in the United States: Sociocultural context for mental health and developmental psychopathology. In A. J. Sameroff, M. Lewis, & S. M. Miller (Eds.), *Handbook of developmental psychopathology* (2nd ed., pp. 177–195). Dordrecht, The Netherlands: Kluwer Academic Publishers.

Gonzales, N. A., Dumka, L. E., Mauricio, A. M., & Germán, M. (2007). Building bridges: Strategies to promote academic and psychological resilience for adolescents of Mexican origin. In J. E. Lansford, K. Deater-Deckard, & M. H. Bornstein (Eds.), *Immigrant families in contemporary society. Duke series in child development and public policy* (pp. 268–286). New York: Guilford Press.

Hardway, C., & Fuligni, A. J. (2006). Dimensions of family connectedness among adolescents with Mexican, Chinese, and European backgrounds. *Developmental Psychology, 42*(6), 1246–1258.

Hernandez, D. J. (2004). Demographic change and the life circumstances of immigrant families. *The Future of Children, 14*(2), 17–47.

Hogg, M. A. (2003). Social identity. In M. R. L. J. P. Tangney (Ed.), *Handbook of self and identity* (pp. 462–479). New York: Guilford Press.

Hughes, D., & Chen, L. (1997). When and what parents tell children about race: An examination of race-related socialization among African American families. *Applied Developmental Science, 1*(4), 200–214.

Huynh, V. W., & Fuligni, A. J. (2008). Ethnic socialization and the academic adjustment of adolescents from Mexican, Chinese, and European backgrounds. *Developmental Psychology, 44*(4), 1202–1208.

Kiang, L., & Fuligni, A. J. (2009). Ethnic identity and family processes among adolescents from Latin American, Asian, and European backgrounds. *Journal of Youth and Adolescence, 38*, 228–241.

Kiang, L., Witkow, M., Baldelomar, O., & Fuligni, A. J. (2010). Change in ethnic identity across the high school years among adolescents with Latin American, Asian, and European backgrounds. *Journal of Youth and Adolescence, 39*, 683–693.

Kiang, L., Yip, T., Gonzales-Backen, M., Witkow, M., & Fuligni, A. J. (2006). Ethnic identity and the daily psychological well being of adolescents with Chinese and Mexican backgrounds. *Child Development, 27*, 1338–1350.

Lagrand, W. K., Visser, C. A., Hermens, W. T., Niessen, G. W. M., Vergeugt, R. W. A., Wolbink, G. J., et al. (1999). C-reactive protein as a cardiovascular risk factor: more than an epiphenomenon? *Circulation, 100*, 96–102.

Lorr, M., & McNair, D. M. (1971). *The profile of mood states manual*. San Francisco: Educational and Industrial Testing Service.

Mroczek, D. K., & Kolarz, C. M. (1998). The effect of age on positive and negative affect: A developmental perspective on happiness. *Journal of Personality and Social Psychology, 75*(5), 1333–1349.

Phinney, J. S. (1990). Ethnic identity in adolescents and adults: Review of research. *Psychological Bulletin, 108*(3), 499–514.

Phinney, J. S., & Rosenthal, D. A. (1992). Ethnic identity in adolescence: Process, context, and outcome. In G. R. Adams, T. P. Gullotta, & R. Montemayor (Eds.), *Adolescent identity formation. Advances in adolescent development* (Vol. 4, pp. 145–172). Thousand Oaks, CA: Sage Publications, Inc.

Ramirez, R. R., & de la Cruz, G. P. (2002). The Hispanic Population in the United States: March 2002. Current Population Reports, pp. 20–545. Washington DC: US Census Bureau.

Ranjit, N., Diez-Roux, A., Shea, S., Cushman, M., Seeman, T. E., Jackson, S. A., et al. (2007). Psychosocial factors and inflammation in the multi-ethnic study of atherosclerosis. *Archives of Internal Medicine, 167*, 174–181.

Reeves, T., & Bennett, C. (2003). *The Asian and Pacific Islander population in the United States: March 2002*. Washington, DC: U.S. Census Bureau.

Ryan, R. M., & Deci, E. L. (2001). On happiness and human potentials: A review of research on hedonic and eudaimonic well-being. *Annual Review of Psychology, 52*, 141–166.

Ryff, C. D. (1989). Happiness is everything, or is it? Explorations on the meaning of psychological well-being. *Journal of Personality and Social Psychology, 57*(6), 1069–1081.

Ryff, C. D. (1995). Psychological well-being in adult life. *Current Directions in Psychological Science, 4*(4), 99–104.

Ryff, C. D., Keyes, C. L. M., & Hughes, D. L. (2003). Status inequalities, perceived piscrimination, and eudaimonic well-being: Do the challenges of minority life hone purpose and growth? *Journal of Health and Social Behavior, 44*(3), 275–291.

Sellers, R. M., Rowley, S. A. J., Chavous, T. M., Shelton, J. N., & Smith, M. A. (1997). Multidimensional inventory of black identity: A preliminary investigation of reliability and construct validity. *Journal of Personality and Social Psychology, 73*(4), 805–815.

Tajfel, H., & Turner, J. (2001). An integrative theory of intergroup conflict. In M. A. Hogg & D. Abrams (Eds.), *Relations: Essential readings. Key readings in social psychology* (pp. 94–109). New York: Psychology Press.

Telzer, E. H., & Fuligni, A. J. (2009a). Daily family assistance and the psychological well being of adolescents from Latin American, Asian, and European backgrounds. *Developmental Psychology, 45,* 1177–1189.

Telzer, E. H., & Fuligni, A. J. (2009b). A longitudinal daily diary study of family assistance and academic achievement among adolescents from Mexican, Chinese, and European backgrounds. *Journal of Youth and Adolescence, 38,* 560–571.

Zhou, M., Lee, J., Vallejo, J. A., Tofoya-Estrada, R., & Xiong, Y. S. (2008). Success attained, deterred, and denied: Divergent pathways to social mobility in Los Angeles' new second generation. *The Annals of the American Academic of Political and Social Science, 620,* 37–61.

The Beginnings of Mental Health Disparities: Emergent Mental Disorders Among Indigenous Adolescents

Les B. Whitbeck

Indigenous people (American Indian/Alaska Natives; AI/AN) make up the smallest ethnic group in the United States comprising about 1.5% of the population (4.3 million people, Ogunwole, 2006), yet they rank higher in health disparities than any other ethnic group. The current life expectancy for an Indigenous person born today is nearly 5 years shorter than that of the general population (72.3 vs. 76.9 years). They are nearly six times more likely to die from alcoholism then are other Americans, five times more likely to die from tuberculosis, three times more likely to die from diabetes, and three times more likely to die from unintentional injuries, homicide or suicide (Indian Health Service, 1992). Indigenous children are more than twice as likely to die in the first 4 years of life than are other American children. Yet, many national health surveillance reports do not even include categories for Indigenous people.

There are several reasons for the absence of an American Indian/Alaska Native category in many national health reports. Foremost is the challenge of obtaining nationally representative samples of such a diverse population. Although researchers and epidemiologists treat Indigenous people as a single ethnic category, there are 562 federally recognized tribes (Bureau of Indian Affairs, 2002) and about 226 tribes that are not recognized by the federal government (Manataka American Indian Council, 2009). These tribes include over 200 distinct languages and vary widely in economies, traditional ways, and spiritual beliefs. Not only are Indigenous cultures ethnically diverse, they are geographically dispersed. About one-third of Indigenous people currently reside on reservations or federal trust lands (Ogunwole, 2006). Tribal reservations tend to be rural, small, and often geographically isolated which makes their inclusion in community samples difficult.

Moreover, after years of exploitation by researchers, many tribal leaders maintain a healthy skepticism about engaging in research activities. Current research ethics stipulate the need for tribal council resolutions for studies on reservations, and for some Indigenous nations, this includes tribal members who live off reservations as

L.B. Whitbeck (✉)
Department of Sociology, University of Nebraska-Lincoln, Lincoln, NE 68588-0324, USA
e-mail: lwhitbeck2@unlnotes.unl.edu

G. Carlo et al. (eds.), *Health Disparities in Youth and Families*, Nebraska
Symposium on Motivation 57, DOI 10.1007/978-1-4419-7092-3_6,
© Springer Science+Business Media, LLC 2011

well. The lengthy, often uncertain approval process complicates the development of large random samples across multiple cultures. Most of our national estimates of Indigenous health care and disease prevalence are from Indian Health Service (IHS) data. However, even these data are not truly representative in that IHS serves less than one-half of Indigenous people living in the US.

Disparities in mental health between Indigenous people and other ethnic groups exceed those of physical health primarily because we know so little about Indigenous mental illness or the best ways to treat it. First, we are not sure exactly what "mental health" means in Indigenous cultures (Thompson, 1996; Trimble, Manson, Dinges, & Medicine, 1984). Concepts of mental illness and symptoms of emotional discomfort may not translate well between European and Indigenous cultures. For example, Manson has pointed out that the terms "depressed" and "anxious" are absent from some Indigenous languages (Manson, Shore, & Bloom, 1985).

Second, there has been only one large population study of mental and substance use disorders among Indigenous peoples and it covered only the Northern Plains and Southwest cultures (Beals et al., 2005; Manson, Beals, Klein, & Croy, 2005; Spicer et al., 2003). Even less mental health research pertaining to Indigenous children exists. To our knowledge, there have been only three diagnostic studies in the past decade that provide information about Indigenous children in the US. The Great Smokey Mountain Study (GSMS) contained a subsample of 323 Cherokee children aged 9, 11 and 13 years (Costello, Farmer, Angold, Burns, & Erkanli, 1997). The prevalence of mental disorder among the Indigenous children (17%) was similar to or lower than that of non-Indigenous study children (19%) with the exception of substance use or dependence (1.2% vs. 0.1%). The second diagnostic study was a school-based sample of 109 Northern Plains adolescents aged 13–17 years where 15% of the adolescents met criteria for one mental disorder and 13% met criteria for two or more disorders (Beals et al., 1997). The third study is the only longitudinal diagnostic study of Indigenous children and the subject of this chapter. The 746 tribally enrolled children were screened for mental disorders using the Diagnostic Interview Schedule for Children-Revised (DISC-R) at ages 10–12 years and at ages 13–15 years (Whitbeck, Hoyt, & Johnson, 2006; Whitbeck, Yu, Johnson, Hoyt, & Walls, 2008).

Accounting for Cultural Contexts of Development

The theoretical model that guides this program of research takes two types of risk and protective factors into account (Fig. 1): (1) general factors identified in research with majority youth that are likely to have similar effects among young people regardless of culture, and (2) culturally specific factors that may affect only children from a particular ethnic group. Risk and protective factors occur in multiple domains: individual, family, school and peer groups, and community. The individual domain includes familial health risks, developmental processes such as puberty (which may interact with prior risks), adolescent temperament (e.g., sensation seeking, risk-taking, irritability), psychological characteristics (e.g., depressive

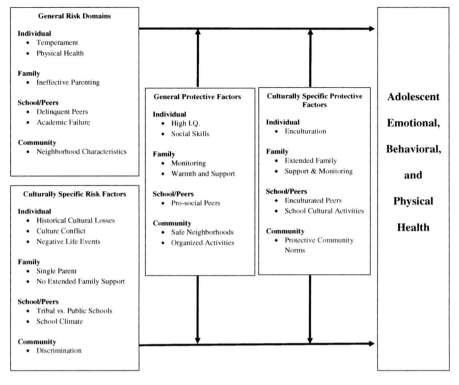

Fig. 1 Theoretical model of research program

symptoms, anxiety), unique life histories (e.g., negative life events, trauma), and specific talents or capabilities. The family domain is the basic socializing context that fosters social skills, monitors behaviors, provides nurturance, and models adult behaviors. As children move through adolescence, experiences outside the family become increasingly influential. School, peer group, and community contexts such as neighborhood characteristics, economic opportunities, and risk of violence have been shown to have major effects on adolescent development (Sampson & Laub, 1993). The model assumes the effects of risk factors are not simply additive; rather, risks can interact with one another to influence adolescent outcomes.

Each of these domains has cultural variations in actual circumstances and the ways the contexts are viewed and experienced. A general theoretical model of adolescent risk will miss these variations and fail to explain a significant proportion of the variance of risk factors on health outcomes unique to specific cultures. Our guiding theoretical model includes culturally specific risk factors, such as perceived discrimination, acculturation, and beliefs, as well as cultural variations in factors such as family influence, family stressors and strengths, and community characteristics.

Risks are influenced by multiple factors, some of which amplify the risk factors (e.g., school leaving) while others may moderate or ameliorate the risk factor (e.g., school adjustment, special talents, caring adults). Indigenous adolescents experience specific risk and protective factors associated with their status that general risk models ignore. For example, among most Indigenous people traditional norms of sharing, respect for others, obligation to family and community conflict with European American individualist norms of competition and accumulation of wealth and power. To be successful and "noticed" at school the child must meet competitive and individualist standards. Those who ascribe to traditional norms of not putting oneself forward or openly competing may become "invisible" in a mixed ethnic classroom. But, if they adopt the European American norms and enact them at home, they may be considered selfish, boastful, and disrespectful of others.

At the same time minority cultures offer specific protective factors to their children such as supporting and monitoring extended family systems, and the protective effects of enculturation (e.g., traditional spirituality, traditional practices, and cultural identity) (Vega, Gil, & Zimmerman, 1993; Whitbeck, Chen, Hoyt, & Adams, 2004; Williams, Spencer, & Jackson, 1999). In summary, this theoretical model hypothesizes that disparities in minority health outcomes cannot be fully understood or addressed without a culturally inclusive approach committed to identifying and recognizing the importance of risk and protective factors tied to cultural context.

Culturally Specific Risk Factors

In this chapter we focus on several culturally specific aspects of Indigenous child development: individual experiences of negative life events, enculturation, aspects of the family context such as maternal mental health, family monitoring and warmth and supportiveness, peer and school influences, and the community influence of discrimination. We begin by describing the unique cultural context in which the adolescents are growing up.

The Developmental Contexts of Reservations/Reserves

Growing up on a US reservation or a Canadian First Nations reserve represents a distinctive developmental context historically and socially. If the indigenous nation was lucky enough not to be completely removed from their home territory, reservations/reserves represent the remnant "homeland." However, this "homeland" often occupies the least productive, least desirable area of what was once their vast territory. As a social context, reservations/reserves are at once a symbol of what was and the representation of what has occurred. The land represents a revered past, yet the histories of some reservations/reserves are filled with stories of epidemics, corrupt government agents, food shortages, boarding schools, and repression. Simply living on reservations/reserves can be a reminder of ethnic cleansing, broken promises, continual encroachment on tribal lands, and continuing pressures of assimilation. At the same time, a reservation/reserve may be a refuge from discrimination and the land a symbol of the living culture. They hold sacred places, and remain the repository of cultural knowledge.

Social problems endemic to reservation life have been well documented (Indian Health Service, 2009; Sandefur, Rindfuss, & Cohen, 1996). Reservation American Indian adolescents are exposed to chronic economic disadvantage (Gregory, Abello, & Johnson, 1996; Trosper, 1996). For example, nearly one-fourth of the caretakers of the study adolescents were unemployed. Only about one-third of children currently lived with their biological father and more than one-fourth (28.5%) of the single income households reported incomes of $10,000 or less as did 12.9% of the dual earner households. This is $4,000 less than the DHHS poverty guidelines for a family of two and $11,200 less than the cut-off for a family of four (Department of Health and Human Services, 2009).

Reservation children are often exposed to violence and other stressful life events (Bachman, 1992). Twenty percent of the caretakers from participating reservations/reserves reported violence towards themselves or a household member in the past 12 months, and of these, 60.6% reported violence on two or more occasions. The caretaking adults in the study were twice as apt to have lost a family member or close friend to death than were adults in the general population (57.6% vs. 28%), about three times more likely to have a family member with a serious illness or injury (33.5% vs. 12.1%), and twice as likely to have been victimized by crime (10.9% vs. 5.1%) (see Hobson, Dulunas, & Kesic, 2001 for general population comparisons to our data).

Family Contexts

Parental mental health problems such as depression and substance abuse are strongly associated with ineffective parenting (Billings & Moos, 1983; Conger, 1997; Conger et al., 1991; Loeber, Farrington, Stouthamer-Loeber, & Van Kammern, 1998; Ovaschel, 1983). The children in the present study are at particular risk for nonoptimal parenting attributable to mental health or substance abuse problems. To place rates for mental disorder among the study parents/caretakers in perspective, rates for lifetime diagnoses were compared to national prevalence rates by selecting those in the same age categories (i.e., 17–54 years) from the US population in the National Comorbidity Survey (NCS). We also compared the rates for the Northern Midwest sample to those of AI-SUPERPFP (ages 15–54 years). (Note: For a discussion on the limitations of these comparisons and the potential for method variance between studies, see Beals et al., 2005; Whitbeck, Hoyt, Chen & Johnson, 2006).

The study adult fathers/male caretakers (54.7%) were four times more likely to meet lifetime criteria for alcohol abuse than were NCS adults (13.1%). They were five times more likely to meet lifetime criteria for alcohol abuse than males from the AI-SUPERPFP Southwest cultures (11.2%), and four times more likely than males from the Northern Plains cultures (12.8%). Differences in rates of lifetime alcohol dependence were not as great. Twenty-seven percent of study fathers/male caretakers met lifetime criteria for alcohol dependence compared to 22.6% of their NCS counterparts, 31.1% of AI-SUPERPFP Southwest males and 30.5% of Northern

Plains males. The prevalence of lifetime alcohol abuse among the mothers/female caretakers (47.7%) was more than six times that of their NCS counterparts (7.2%), nine times that for AI-SUPERPFP Southwest females (5.1%) and four times that for Northern Plains females (10.3%). Although similar to women in the Northern Plains (20.5%), the study mothers/female caretakers (19.1%) were twice as likely as NCS females (9.1%) and Southwest females (8.7%) to meet lifetime criteria for alcohol dependence. Rates of lifetime major depressive episode (MDE) among the mothers/female caretakers (20.7%) were very similar to those for NCS females (22.1%). However, the study women were more likely to meet lifetime criteria for MDE than Southwest (14.3%) or Northern Plains women (10.3%). The study fathers/male caretakers reported lower rates of MDE (9.6%) than did their counterparts in the NCS (13.7%), but rates for MDE were very similar to Southwest (9.8%) and Northern Plains (7.2%) males in the AI-SUPERPFP study.

"Family" vs. "Parental" Influence

Researchers who mistakenly assume that Indigenous family influence occurs only in the context of the parent-child relationship will miss potentially important sources of influence on children. Focusing on "parenting" ignores extended family members who may provide some or all of the functions included in such measures as parental warmth and support, approval, monitoring, and even discipline. To account for this, we asked the children who performed "parenting" functions in their lives. For example, when we administered our measure of monitoring, we asked seven monitoring questions such as: "In a usual day, how often does someone in your family know where you are?" Then we asked: "Now thinking about the questions I just asked you, who in your family would be the one to know the *most* about where you are and what you are doing away from home?" This was followed by a series of questions: "Would anyone else in your family be likely to know where you are and what you are doing away from home?" The interviewer would allow up to five iterations or would stop when they child said no one else performed that family function.

Peer Contexts

There is concern that peer pressure may be especially pertinent to American Indian young people. For example, local norms may portray alcohol and tobacco use as indicative of adulthood (Topper, 1980). Moreover, active refusal or rejection of alcohol and drug using friends may be viewed as rude and confrontational by the culture (Beauvais, 1980; Leland, 1980; Weibel, 1982). Many of the study adolescents had close friends who were engaging in problem behaviors. For example, at ages 12–14 years (Wave 3), 43% of the adolescents reported that at least one of their three best friends smoked cigarettes, one-third had at least one best friend who drank alcohol, 37% had at least one best friend who was not getting along with his/her parents, and 44% had at least one best friend who had been in trouble with the police.

School Adjustment

Teenagers spend the majority of their week days at school. Overtime, those who view school as supportive, their classes meaningful, and their teachers caring fare better socially and show better emotional adjustment. They also are more resilient in the face of adversities (Roeser, Eccles, & Sameroff, 2000). Positive relationships with teachers are associated with higher self-esteem (Hoge, Smit, & Hanson, 1990), and fewer risk behaviors (Steinberg, 1996). There is evidence that Indigenous adolescents respond to school environments that are supportive and culturally attuned (Lysne & Levy, 1997). Among the students in this study, positive school adjustment declined over time among those who attended public schools on or off the reservation/reserve but remained stable across time for those in tribal schools. Moreover, the negative effects of discrimination on school adjustment were greater for students in public schools compared to those in tribal schools (Crawford, Cheadle, & Whitbeck, 2009).

Discrimination

There is a rapidly emerging literature pertaining to discrimination-induced stress affects on physical and mental health among minority groups (Kessler, Mickelson, & Williams, 1999; Krieger & Sidney, 1996; Williams & Williams-Morris, 2000; Williams, Yu, & Jackson, 1997). Evidence is accumulating that discrimination functions similarly to other psychological stressors (Dion, Dion, & Pak, 1992; Thompson, 1996; Williams et al., 1999) and that it is a primary contributor to psychological distress among minority people. Kessler and colleagues rank it with major negative life events such as the death of a loved one, divorce or job loss and suggest that "the conjunction of high prevalence and strong impact would mean that discrimination is among the most important of all the stressful experiences that have been implicated as causes of mental health problems" (Kessler et al., 1999, p. 224).

Even when very young, many of the study adolescents had experienced discrimination. About one-half (45.2%) of the 10–12 year old children reported that other kids have made insulting comments based on ethnicity, and about one-third (31%) have had racial slurs yelled at them. More than one-third (38.3%) of the children believe that Indigenous children are disciplined at school differently than European American children. Fourteen percent believe they are treated differently by school bus drivers. Ten percent dreaded going to school because of their treatment and 7% dreaded riding the bus to and from school.

Enculturation as a Protective Factor

"Enculturation" refers to the degree to which individuals are embedded in their cultures as manifested by practicing the traditional culture and self-reported cultural identity (Zimmerman, Ramirez, Washienko, Walter, & Dyer, 1998). For several decades (and historically among most tribal elders) there has been a movement to use traditional cultural knowledge in various treatment and educational settings. Although early studies attempting to empirically demonstrate the effectiveness of cultural identity and traditional culture showed mixed results at best (Beauvais, 1998), as measures improved evidence began to accumulate that traditional cultural ways and beliefs can be therapeutic. The most compelling evidence has come from the application of traditional beliefs, values, and practices in alcohol treatment programs (e.g., Gray & Nye, 2001; Herman-Stahl, Spencer, & Duncan, 2003; Moncher, Holden, & Trimble, 1990; Noe, Fleming, & Manson, 2003; Spicer, Novins, Mitchell, & Beals, 2003; Torres-Stone, Whitbeck, Chen, Johnson, & Olson, 2006). Along with numerous researchers, we believe that enculturation is a resiliency factor that may protect against conduct problems, depression, suicide, and substance abuse among adolescents or serve as an important therapeutic factor in treatment programs.

The Longitudinal Study

Community Based Participatory Research with Indigenous People

The data used in this study are part of a longitudinal lagged sequential study currently underway on four Indigenous reservations in the Northern Midwest and four Canadian First Nation reserves. Several of the reserves are classified as "remote" in that they are considerable distances from even small towns and are accessed by non-paved roads, by boat, over ice in winter, or by airplane. The reserves and reservations included in this sample share a common cultural tradition and language with minor regional variations in dialects. The sample is representative of one the most populous Indigenous cultures in the United States and Canada. The long range purpose of the longitudinal study is to identify culturally specific resilience and risk factors that affect children's well-being and to then use the information to guide the development of culturally-based interventions.

The project was designed in partnership with the participating reservations and reserves. Prior to the application funding, the research team was invited to work on these reservations/reserves and tribal resolutions supporting the study were obtained. As part of our agreement to work together, the researchers promised that participating reservations/reserves would be kept confidential in published reports. On each participating reservation/reserve, an advisory board was appointed by the tribal council. The advisory boards were responsible for advice on handling difficult personnel problems, advising on questionnaire development, reading reports for respectful writing, and assuring that published reports protected the identity of the respondents and the culture. Upon advisory board approval of the questionnaires, the study procedures and questionnaires were submitted for review by the university Institutional Review Board for approval.

All participating staff on the reservations were approved by the advisory board and are either tribal members or, in a few cases, non-members who are spouses of tribal members. To ensure quality of data collection, all the interviewers underwent special training for conducting computer-assisted personal interviewing. The training included practice interviews and feedback sessions regarding interview quality. In addition, all of the interviewers completed a required human subject's protection training that emphasized the importance of confidentiality and taught procedures to maintain the confidentiality of data.

Participants

At the beginning of the project, each reservation/reserve provided a list of families of enrolled children aged 10–12 years who lived on or proximate to (within 50 miles) the reservation or reserve. We attempted to contact all families with a child within the specified age range. Families were recruited with a personal visit by an Indigenous interviewer explained the project to them. They were then presented with a traditional gift and invited to participate. If they agreed to be interviewed, each family member received $40 for their time when the interviews were completed. Study adolescents and at least one of their adult caretakers were interviewed annually over the course of the study.

At Wave 1, the majority (97%) of the 746 youths interviewed were 10–12 years old; however, because of recruitment errors and birthdays between recruitment and interview dates, a small number of youth were aged 9 or 13 at Wave 1. The overall response rate for all sites at baseline was 79.4%. Subsequent retention rates were 95% at Wave 2, 93% for Wave 3, and 90% for Wave 4 of data collection.

Measures

As best we were able, the measures used in our analyses parallel those in our theoretical model of risk and protective factors.

Risk Factors

Mother/female caretaker major depressive episode was measured with a dichotomous variable indicating if female caretakers met lifetime criteria for major depressive episode (MDE) at Wave 1 based on the University of Michigan Composite International Diagnostic Interview (UM-CIDI). The UM-CIDI was derived from the Diagnostic and Statistical Manual-III-R (DSM-III-R) criteria and represents the University of Michigan revision of the World Health Organization CIDI used in the National Comorbidity Survey (NCS, Kessler, 1994a, 1994b). The CIDI, on which the UM-CIDI is based is a well-established diagnostic instrument that has shown excellent inter-rater reliability, test-retest reliability, and validity for the diagnoses used in this study. The UM-CIDI has been used extensively with trained interviewers who are not clinicians. The version used in this study included cultural modifications similar to those in the AI-SUPERPFP (Beals et al., 2005). Eighteen percent of female caretakers met criteria for lifetime MDE.

Mother/female caretaker lifetime substance use disorder was measured with a dichotomous variable indicating if caretakers met UM-CIDI lifetime criteria for at least one of three substance abuse disorders (SUD): alcohol abuse, alcohol dependence, or drug abuse at Wave 1. A value of 1 indicated that female caretakers met criteria for at least one SUD. Sixty-five percent of female caretakers met lifetime criteria for at least one SUD.

Adolescent negative life events were measured with a ten-item summed scale at all three waves. The adolescents were asked whether any of the following 10 things had happened to them during the past 12 months.

1. Friend died
2. Close relative died
3. Pet died
4. Close friend moved away
5. Someone close to you got sick or hurt
6. Sibling got into serious trouble at school
7. Sibling got into serious trouble with police
8. You were seriously sick or hurt
9. Elder passed on
10. Parents separated or divorced.

The scores were then averaged across the three waves.

Deviant peer affiliations were measured with a five-item summed scale at all three waves. The adolescents indicated how many of their three best friends engaged in the following behaviors: smoking cigarettes, drinking alcohol, poor parent relations, trouble with school, and trouble with police. Scores were then averaged across the three waves.

Perceived discrimination was measured using a nine-item summed and meaned scale assessing perceived discrimination in the community and school at each wave. Items included whether students had been insulted, disrespected, ignored, threatened, or treated different by police, school staff, community members, and peers. Variables were recoded so a higher score indicates experiencing more discrimination (0 = never, 1 = a few times, 2 = many times). Scores were then averaged across the three waves. Alphas ranged from 0.81 to 0.84 across all three waves.

Protective Factors

Family monitoring was measured with a five-item summed scale at all three waves. The adolescents were asked to indicate how many people know where they are and what they are doing when they are away from home. Respondents checked all that applied to the following categories: mother, father, siblings, aunt/uncle, and grandparent. The number of "family monitors" was then averaged across the three waves.

Family warmth and supportiveness was similarly measured with a five item sum scale at all three waves. The adolescents were asked to indicate how many people listened to and talked with them about positive choices, rules, problems, and decisions. Respondents checked all that applied to the following categories: mother, father, siblings, aunt/uncle, and grandparent. The number of warm and supportive family members were then averaged across the three waves.

Positive school adjustment was measured with a seven item sum scale at each wave assessing general attitudes towards school. Alphas ranged from 0.73 to 0.76 across all three waves. Items assessed if students liked school, did well in school, tried hard at school, felt grades were important, got along with teachers, did well in hard subjects, and felt teachers saw them as good students. Variables were recoded so that a higher score indicates more positive adjustment. Scores were then averaged across the three waves.

Cultural intervention. Cultural intervention was measured with a four item sum scale at each wave assessing if youth has participated in the following activities in the previous year.

1. Participated in a sweat
2. Gone to a traditional healer
3. Sought advice from a spiritual advisor
4. Used traditional medicine.

Scores were then averaged across the three waves.

Control Variables

Adolescent's *age* was measured using a continuous variable at Wave 1. *Gender* was controlled by a dummy variable where 1 = female and 0 = male. Fifty-two percent of our sample was male. *Family per capita Income* was measured by household per capital yearly income. Families were asked to indicate whether their overall household incomes were above or below $25,000 in the past year. Two additional questions narrowed these responses to within $10,000 ranges. The midpoints of each of these ranges were used to sum the two variables, which were then divided by the number of people living within the household at least 50% of the time. *Remote* location was measured using a dichotomous variable (0,1) where a score of 1 indicates that families on or near a remote Canadian reserve.

The Beginnings of Mental Health Disparities

At an average age of about 11 years, 25.6% of the Indigenous children met diagnostic criteria for at least one mental disorder and 9.2% met criteria for two or more disorders. By the time the adolescents had reached an average of 14.3 years, 44.8%

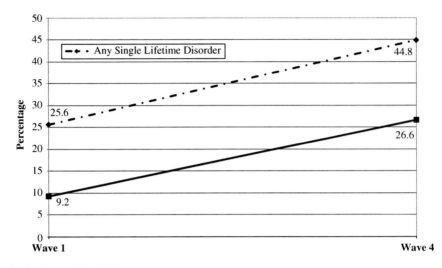

Fig. 2 Comorbidity lifetime

met criteria for a single disorder and 26.6% met criteria for two or more disorders (Fig. 2).

These numbers correspond to the lifetime prevalence for psychiatric disorders in the National Comorbidity Survey Replication (NCS-R) for adults aged 18 years and older, 46.4% single diagnosis; 27.7% two or more diagnoses (Kessler, Berglund, Demler, Jin, & Walters, 2005). In the American Indian Service Utilization, Psychiatric Epidemiology, Risk and Protective Factors Project (AI-SUPERPFP), prevalence rates for meeting lifetime criteria for at least one mental disorder among respondents aged 15–54 years were 41.9% for Southwest Indigenous cultures and 44.5% for Northern Plains cultures (Beals et al., 2005). These adolescent prevalence rates also correspond to those of the adolescents' adult caretakers, 43% for a single disorder and 31.6% for two or more disorders (Whitbeck, Hoyt, Chen, & Johnson, 2006).

The increase in mental disorders in these few short years of adolescent development was dramatic. The prevalence of lifetime alcohol abuse increased from 1.1 to 13.8% and lifetime alcohol dependence increased from 0.5 to 7.2% (Fig. 3).

Lifetime nicotine dependence increased from 1.7 to 9.5%, lifetime marijuana increased from 0.6 to 8.0%, and lifetime marijuana dependence went from 1.4 to 12.4% (Fig. 4). Meeting lifetime criteria for any substance abuse disorder increased from 3.2 to 27.2% (Fig. 5). The 12-month substance use disorder prevalence for Indigenous adolescents was 25.5%, nearly three times that reported in the National Survey on Drug Use and Health (9.4% of adolescents 12 years and older) (Substance Abuse and Mental Health Services Administration, 2006).

Twelve-month major depressive episode increased from 3.2 to 7.8% (Fig. 6) well within the expected 1.6–8.9% range for adolescents of this age (Angold & Costello, 2001). Among externalizing disorders lifetime conduct disorder increased

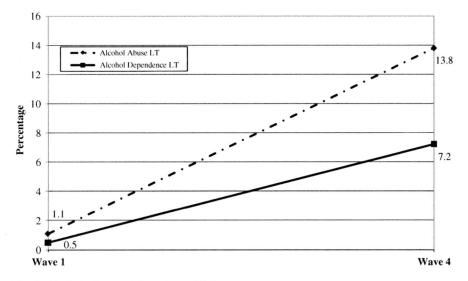

Fig. 3 Alcohols abuse and dependence-lifetime

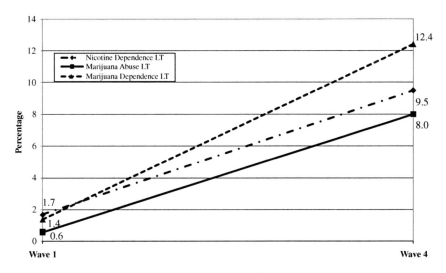

Fig. 4 Nicotine and marijuana abuse and dependance-lifetime

from 12.3 to 23.4%, (Fig. 7). Estimates of conduct disorder among children aged 8–16 years in Western industrialized countries range between 5 and 10% (Angold & Costello, 2001). The rates among Indigenous children were more than twice the highest expected rate.

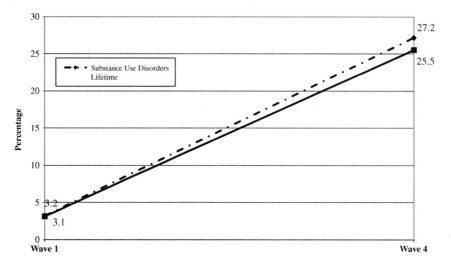

Fig. 5 Any substance use disorder-12 month and lifetime

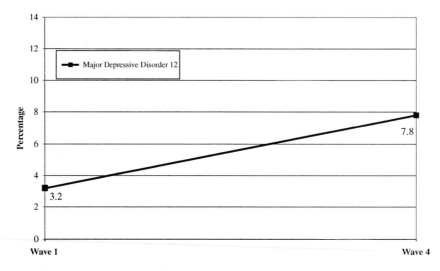

Fig. 6 Major depressive disorders-12 month

Antecedents of Early On-Set Conduct Disorder and Substance Use Disorders

To make optimal use of our longitudinal data, we dropped all of the cases where the adolescents met diagnostic criteria at year one and focused on those who developed a mental disorder between years one and four of the study. This allowed us to evaluate factors that contributed to emergent mental disorders. We focused on conduct

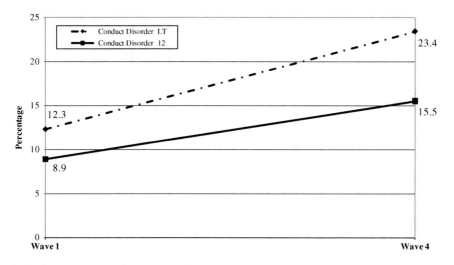

Fig. 7 Conduct disorder lifetime and 12 month

disorder and substance use disorders because they were so highly prevalent among the Indigenous young people.

Problem behavior theory suggests that adolescent problem behaviors are highly interrelated and tend to co-occur (Costa, Jessor, Donovan, & Fortenberry, 1995; Jessor & Jessor, 1977). They often are so strongly correlated that we can lose valuable information when they are all included in a single regression equation. One or two particularly robust correlates may reduce the contributions of collinear variables to non-significance yet these variables contribute to the explained variance. For this reason we begin our investigation with regression equations that contain only the control variables and stepped in variable domains of interest.

Antecedents of Conduct Disorder

The first set of regression models (Table 1) focus on the onset of conduct disorder by Wave 4 of the study when the adolescents averaged about age 14 years (range = 12–15 years). The first regression equation contained only the control variables: gender, age, per capita family income, and whether the adolescent was from a rural or remote reservation or Canadian reserve. Only family per capita income was statistically significant, decreasing the odds of meeting lifetime criteria for CD by 7% for each additional $1,000 of family income.

In Model 2, mother/female caretaker lifetime major depressive disorder and substance use disorder were added into the equation with the control variables. Maternal/female caretaker's lifetime major depressive episode increased the odds of their child meeting criteria for CD 70% ($p \leq 0.10$). In Model 3, adolescents' perceptions of the number of family members who monitored their behaviors and

Table 1 Logistic regression predicting lifetime CD-W4

	Model 1		Model 2		Model 3		Model 4		Model 5		Model 6		Model 7		Model 8	
	B	Exp(b)	B	Exp(b)	B	Exp(b)	B	Exp(b)	B	Exp(b)	B	Exp(b)	B	Exp(b)	B	Exp(b)
Female	-0.14	0.87	-0.17	0.85	-0.15	0.86	-0.16	0.85	-0.19	0.83	-0.11	0.90	-0.11	0.90	-0.16	0.85
Age	0.22	1.25	0.22	1.25	0.20	1.22	0.24	1.27	-0.19	0.91	0.20	1.22	0.19	1.21	-0.07	0.93
Family per capita income	**-0.07**	**0.93** *	**-0.07**	**0.94** *	**-0.06**	**0.94** *	-0.05	0.95	-0.03	0.97	-0.06	0.95 †	-0.05	0.95 †	-0.01	0.99
Remote	-0.23	0.79	-0.07	0.93	-0.04	0.67	-0.13	0.87	-0.22	0.80	-0.46	0.63	-0.27	0.76	-0.38	0.68
Major depression-female caretaker			**0.53**	**1.7** †											0.37	1.45
Substance use disorder-female care taker			0.30	1.35											0.10	1.11
Family monitoring					-0.35	0.70									-0.22	0.80
Family warmth and supportiveness					-0.12	0.89									-0.11	0.89
Negative life events							0.26	1.29 ***							0.05	1.05
Peer influence									0.23	1.26 ***					**0.18**	**1.2** ***
Positive school adjustment									-0.24	0.78 *					**-0.25**	**0.78** *
Cultural healing											0.05	1.65 ***			**0.32**	**1.38** †
Discrimination													**1.74**	**5.68** ***	0.70	2.01
Constant	**-3.34**	**0.04** *	**-3.7**	**0.02** *	-2.11	0.12	**-4.36**	**0.01** **	0.37	1.44	**-3.49**	**0.03** *	**-3.5**	**0.03** *	0.32	1.37

* p < 0.05; ** p < 0.01; *** p < 0.001; † p < 0.10.

who were warm and supportive towards them were non-significant. In Model 4, adolescents' stressful life events increased the odds of meeting criteria for lifetime CD by 29% with only the control variables in the equation. Associating with delinquent peers increased the odds of lifetime CD by 26% and positive school attitudes reduced the odds of CD by 22% for each average unit increase in the measures (Model 5). Meeting lifetime criteria for CD increased the odds of cultural intervention 65% for each average unit increase in the measure. Adolescents who were manifesting problem behaviors were more likely to talk with elders and spiritual advisors and engage in other healing activities (Model 6). With only the control variables in the model, adolescents' perceptions of discrimination increased the odds of lifetime CD more than five times for each average unit increase in the measure (Model 7).

With all of the variables in the regression model only affiliation with delinquent peers and positive school adjustment remained statistically significant. Associating with delinquent peers increased the odds of lifetime CD by 20% for each average increase in the number of delinquent friends. Positive school adjustment reduced the odds of CD by 22% for each average unit increase in the measure. Cultural healing was positively associated with meeting criteria for CD ($p \leq 0.10$).

Antecedents of Substance Use Disorders

We followed the same procedures for evaluating antecedents to meeting lifetime criteria for any substance use disorder (SUD) by Wave 4 of the study (Table 2). Among the control variables (Model 1), being female increased the odds of meeting lifetime criteria for SUD by 64%, and for each year of age the odds increased 92%. When mother/female caretaker lifetime major depressive episode and substance use disorder were added to the equation, maternal/female caretaker major depressive episode increased the odds of offspring's SUD by 66% and maternal SUD increased the odds by 0.51% ($p \leq 0.10$). In Model 3 with just the control variables and family influence variables in the model, family monitoring decreased the odds of SUD at Wave 4 by 40% for each additional family monitor. Adolescent negative life events increased the odds of lifetime SUD at Wave 4 by 18% for each average increase in negative events with only the control variables in the model (Model 4). Affiliation with delinquent peers increased the odds of lifetime SUD by 24% and positive school adjustment decreased the odds by 27% for each average unit increase in the measures (Model 5). Adolescents on a pathway towards substance use disorder were 47% more likely to receive some sort of cultural intervention (Model 6), and adolescents who perceived they were being discriminated against were nearly four times more likely to meet lifetime criteria for SUD for each average unit increase in the measure at Wave 4 (Model 7)

With all of the variables in the regression model, females were 71% more likely than males to meet lifetime criteria for any SUD by Wave 4 and for each year of age, the odds of meeting criteria for any SUD increased 50%. Family monitoring remained statistically significant with all of the variables in the model and decreased

Table 2 Logistic regression predicting lifetime SUD-W4

	Model 1		Model 2		Model 3		Model 4		Model 5		Model 6		Model 7		Model 8	
	B	Exp(b)	B	Exp(b)	B	Exp(b)	B	Exp(b)	B	Exp(b)	B	Exp(b)	B	Exp(b)	B	Exp(b)
Female	**0.49**	**1.64** *	**0.48**	**1.62** *	**0.51**	1.66 *	**0.47**	**1.59** *	**0.46**	**1.58** *	**0.54**	**1.72** **	**0.52**	**1.69** **	**0.54**	**1.71** *
Age	**0.65**	**1.92** ***	**0.66**	**1.93** ***	**0.62**	0.92 ***	**0.66**	**1.93** ***	**0.41**	**1.51** **	**0.64**	**1.9** ***	**0.64**	**1.89** ***	**0.41**	**1.5** **
Family per capita income	**-0.09**	**0.92** **	**-0.09**	**0.92** **	**-0.08**	**0.91** **	**-0.08**	**0.93** **	**-0.05**	**0.95** †	**-0.08**	**0.92** **	**-0.08**	**0.92** **	-0.05	0.96
Remote	0.08	1.08	0.28	1.33	-0.10		0.15	1.16	0.18	1.19	-0.08	0.93	0.07	1.07	0.08	1.08
Major depression-female caretaker			**0.51**	**1.66** *											0.38	1.46
Substance use disorder-female care taker			0.40	1.49 †											0.23	1.26
Family monitoring					**-0.52**	**0.60** *									**-0.47**	**0.63** *
Family warmth and supportiveness					-0.03	0.97									0.14	1.15
Negative life events							**0.17**	**1.18** **							-0.06	0.94
Peer influence									**0.22**	**1.24** ***					**0.19**	**1.22** ***
Positive school adjustment									**-0.32**	**0.73** ***					-0.32	0.73 ***
Cultural healing											**0.39**	**1.47** **			0.31	1.37 *
Discrimination													**1.31**	**3.72** **	0.36	1.43
Constant	**-8.12**	**0.00** ***	**-8.57**	**0.00** **	**-6.71**	**0.00** ***	**-8.75**	**0.00** ***	**-4.77**	**0.00** ***	**-8.27**	**0.00** ***	**-8.32**	**0.00** ***	**-4.34**	**0.01** *

$* p < 0.05$; $** p < 0.01$; $*** p < 0.001$; $† p < 0.10$.

the odds of SUD by 37% for each additional family monitor. Affiliating with delinquent peers increased the odds of SUD by 22% and positive school adjustment decreased the odds by 27% for each average increase in the measures. Adolescents on the pathway to SUD were 37% more likely to have some sort of traditional intervention.

Evidence for Malleable Constructs for Interventions

These findings suggest several points of intervention to reduce mental health disparities among Indigenous children. The most important is the window of opportunity for intervention in early adolescence. Clearly, the period between early and mid-adolescence is a critical point for the emergence of mental and substance abuse disorders. As with all children, the first point to intervene is with parents/caretakers. Mothers/female caretakers who were depressed and substance using were more likely to have children who met criteria for CD and SUD. As we have noted elsewhere that rate of lifetime alcohol dependence among the mothers/female caretakers in this study was 18.2%, the rate of lifetime alcohol abuse, 47.7%, and the rate of lifetime drug abuse, 20%. The lifetime prevalence of major depression was 20% (Whitbeck, Hoyt, Chen, & Johnson, 2006). It is critical to evaluate and treat parents as well as children. This is apparent in the strong protective effects for family monitoring against adolescent SUD.

The adolescents are experiencing stressful events at very high rates. Family economic and health disparities take their toll as well. Reducing violence, family disorganization, and loss in the children's lives will make a difference. Also, efforts to engage the children in school will likely pay off in less CD and SUD over time. Prevention efforts also should focus on dealing with discrimination and management of feelings associated with it.

The adolescents who are manifesting problem behaviors are receiving more cultural interventions than those who are not having problems. When you put this finding together with the protective effects we find for enculturation among adults it suggests that the positive effects of enculturation may not show up at these behavioral extremes (i.e. meeting diagnostic criteria) or at this stage of the development of cultural identity (see Phinney & Alipuria, 1990; Phinney, 1989 review). We have found protective effects of enculturation among Indigenous adolescents for symptoms measures of suicide ideation (Yoder, Whitbeck, Hoyt, & LaFromboise, 2006), self-esteem (LaFromboise, Hoyt, Oliver, & Whitbeck, 2006), and for academic achievement (Whitbeck, Hoyt, Stubben, & LaFromboise, 2001), but for adolescents at the behavioral extremes of meeting diagnostic criteria these protective effects are absent but evident in cultural concern or intervention. Whether cultural protective effects emerge as adult identities are established as they have for the children's adult parents/caretakers (e.g., Torres-Stone et al., 2006; Whitbeck, McMorris, Hoyt, Stubben, & LaFromboise, 2002; Whitbeck et al., 2004) is an empirical question.

Creating Partnerships for Empirically Based Culturally Specific Interventions

Nearly every researcher who works with Indigenous people emphasizes the heterogeneity of Native cultures. Still, this is largely ignored by funding agencies, editors, grant reviewers, and epidemiologists who prefer to generalize across Indigenous cultures. Ignoring cultural distinctiveness not only results in poor science, it is disrespectful to generalize across the more than 562 federally recognized tribes (Bureau of Indian Affairs, 2002). These cultures have faced generations of government policies of ethnic cleansing and forced assimilation and continue the struggle to maintain and preserve the traditions, values, and practices that make them unique. Aggregating all Indigenous people into a single ethnic category without regard for cultural differences is more than merely cultural insensitivity; it is yet another manifestation of policies of cultural eradication.

However, there are ways to do respectful, acceptable research with Indigenous people, but the process is labor-intensive, slow, and begins with "small science." Beals and colleagues point out that the process should begin with multiple small separate studies focusing on particular cultures. Measures for key constructs may be adapted and replicated culture by culture creating cumulative knowledge and an empirical foundation for shared constructs for larger studies (Beals, Manson, & Mitchell, 2003). Our community based participatory model (CPBR) for prevention research also proceeds culture by culture. The process may be similar across cultures, and even some of the components of the prevention programs may be similar, however, the language, the values, and traditions on which the prevention is based will be very different. This nation by nation approach is labor intensive, but it acknowledges the unique role of culture and creates active partnerships that increase local ownership, subject response rates, and sustainability. Our model for community based participatory prevention research originates within the culture and takes both general risk and culturally specific risk and protective factors into account (Fig. 8). The critical first stage involves an *invitation* from the community to work with them as an equal partner to create a prevention program. The second stage involves cultural knowledge. Indigenous people have survived one of the longest, most intense, and purposive policies of cultural extermination ever perpetuated on a people. Their cultures are a source of strength. They contain all of the necessary knowledge needed to socialize mentally healthy, substance free children. This knowledge need not be replaced with information and socialization practices from European culture. In Stage 2, researchers work with cultural experts (e.g., elders, services providers, tribal leaders) to identify culturally specific risk and protective factors. Often elders in American Indian cultures know that something works. This knowledge is based on generations of experience, yet it has never been subject to European scientific evaluation. European American researchers must respect this intergenerational cultural knowledge and take it into account.

At Stage 3, these identified risk and protective factors are "translated" into prevention strategies and prevention program components by taking into account research from the majority culture (Stage 3A), existing prevention research with

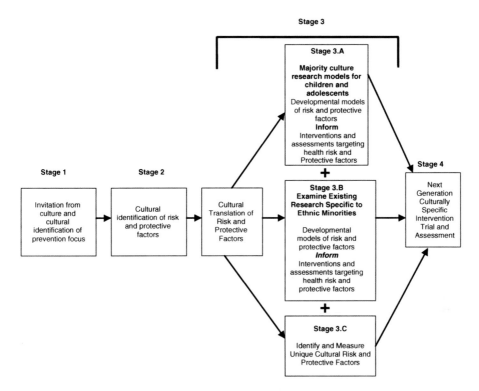

Fig. 8 Model for community based participatory prevention research

other Indigenous cultures (Stage 3B), and information specific to the culture (Stage 3C). European American prevention programs even if loosely adapted may not address critical culturally specific risks or enhance culturally specific protective factors, thus sacrificing power, cultural ownership, and sustainability. The prevention program that results from the research model (Stage 4) will be a blend of cultural knowledge and European knowledge that may be operationalized via culturally specific measures and empirically tested for efficacy.

The problem remains that this and similar approaches are an imperfect fit with European scientific prevention paradigms. Small sample sizes due to small cultural groups or communities reduce statistical power. There are multiple challenges pertaining to randomization including small tightly knit interrelated communities, cultural norms of equality and sharing of resources, lack of strict comparability of control-groups across communities or across reservations/reserves. Even the more populous Indigenous cultures tend to be grouped on small reservations which may differ somewhat economically and geographically.

Perhaps the greatest cultural mismatch with the European research approach is the necessity of progressing slowly and deliberately, always at the pace and comfort level of cultural partners. Working with Indigenous cultures takes time. For example, it may take months to get on the agenda of busy tribal councils just for the initial resolution supporting a research application. The CBPR process involves numerous meetings at each participating reservation/reserve to develop measures and questionnaires, develop the prevention program components, and to jointly oversee the research process. Approval for disseminating research reports can take months prior to journal submission.

In summary, a contributing factor to the persistence of health disparities among Indigenous people has been the ongoing lack of cultural understanding and accommodation between Indigenous people and European American research community. As the motives and approaches of researchers have shifted towards cultural partnerships and the interest in the value of accurate information has increased on the part of Indigenous communities, institutional research norms have not kept up. The next steps will involve working out amenable approaches such as the CBPR model we have outlined that protect and respect Indigenous cultures and engage them in true research partnerships.

Addressing Indigenous Children's Mental Health Disparities

According to a recent Government Accountability Office Report (2005), IHS clinics often lack funds for suitable staff and equipment, are geographically distant and difficult to access, and have long waiting times for specialty services. The IHS appropriated funding provides for only about 55% of costs necessary for "mainstream personal health care services" (Indian Health Service, 2006). Indeed, the 2005 federal budget allocated $1,855 more in per capital health expenditures to the Bureau of Prisons than to IHS ($3,985 vs. $2,130). Indigenous people are even more poorly served for mental health needs than they are for general health care. IHS only allocates about 7% of its funding for mental health and substance abuse treatment (Gone, 2004).

The first explanation usually proffered to account for mental health disparities for Indigenous people is that they under utilize mental health services for reasons of cultural mismatch and distrust. Although most of the evidence for this has been anecdotal (US Department of Health and Human Services, 2001), information from the parents/caretakers of the children in this study indicate that they prefer informal and traditional sources of support for their children's emotional and behavioral problems over institutional sources of care (Walls, Johnson, Whitbeck, & Hoyt, 2006). When asked about the perceived effectiveness of mental health/substance abuse providers for their children, "Counselor on reservation" ranked eighth (32.9%) between sweat lodge (33.2%) and pipe ceremony (30.8%). Nearly all of the cultural interventions ranked higher or equal to institutional interventions (Fig. 9).

Given the interest in traditional sources of support for emotional and behavioral needs, the lack of highly trained Indigenous mental health professionals who understand traditional ways is a major concern. Indigenous professionals not only increase trust, but also are better placed to merge cultural and medical interventions. In 2001, IHS employed about 20 psychiatrists, 60 psychologists, and 110 social workers. Of these, Joseph Gone reports that even given AI/AN hiring preferences, only two

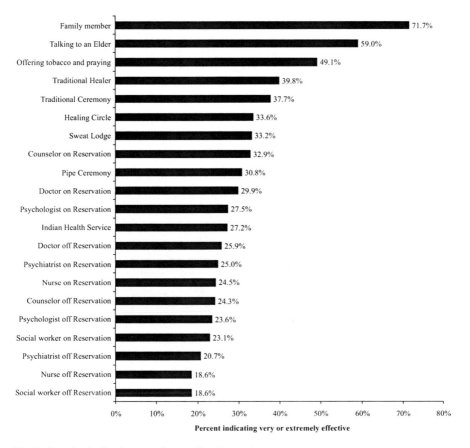

Fig. 9 Perceived effectiveness of mental health services

of the psychiatrists and 17 of the psychologists were AI/AN (Gone, 2003). In the United States the ratios of highly trained mental health professionals are approximately 14 psychiatrists and 28 psychologists per 100,000 people. In comparison IHS has ratios of about two psychiatrists and four psychologists per 100,000 AI/AN people. With this staffing ratio, Gone estimates that the IHS is prepared to meet less than 5% of the mental health needs among AI/AN people.

The situation is not improving. Over the past 30 years there has been little progress in the number of AI/AN medical school applicants. In 1974 there were 127 AI/AN medical school applicants, 30 years later in 2004 this had increased to only 145 compared to 6,734 Asian, 2,802 African American and 2,545 Hispanic applicants (American Association of Medical Colleges, 2005). This count does not reflect the number of applicants interested in specializing in psychiatry. Only 0.1% of clinically trained psychiatrists and 0.6% of psychologists in the US are AI/AN.

Closing the Gap

Health and mental health disparities for Indigenous people are not new. Indeed, they have been ongoing for centuries and have received very little national attention (see Jones, 2006). Calls for changing the funding structure for health care funding are consistently ignored; the Indigenous population is small and lacks political clout. While allocations for Medicaid and Medicare increase dramatically across time, IHS funding has remained essentially flat (Westmoreland & Watson, 2006). Joseph Gone (2004) sums up the current situation:

> Owing to chronic budgetary constraints, recruitment and retention challenges, and routine cultural misunderstanding, the assertion that American Indians and Alaska Natives are "underserved" with regard to mental health care in the United States glibly understates a national travesty that demonstrates an intrinsic but ongoing repudiation of America's longstanding Trust obligations to tribal nations (p. 13).

In a recent editorial for the *Journal of the American Academy of Child and Adolescent Psychiatry*, Barlow and Walkup (2008) pointed out that the need to close the gap between Indigenous children and others is so urgent that we must move beyond basic research "to seek approaches to deploy cost-effective, evidence-based solutions that reflect Indigenous cultural strengths and community will" (p. 843). However, the rapid development of evidence-based prevention and intervention programs will require a new era of cultural understanding and cooperation between Indigenous nations, researchers, and funding agencies. Although some of the agencies understand the nuances of developing CBPR Indigenous prevention and intervention programs the funding process often serves to perpetuate disparities.

Meanwhile, the nations are moving forward on their own with numerous grassroots culturally based prevention efforts. But these grassroots efforts typically lack scientific sophistication both in development (e.g., an empirical foundation) and in the evaluation of the programs (e.g., randomized control groups, statistical power). As our findings suggest, the Nations are already actively intervening at the cultural level, but these efforts need support to demonstrate what works well and what does not. The need is urgent. To address it we make the following recommendations;

1. The case for adequate funding for health and mental programs has been made elsewhere (e.g., Gone, 2004; Westmoreland & Watson, 2006). True progress cannot be achieved without adequate funding.
2. Convening a National Institutes of Health summit on Indigenous health prevention and treatment funding. Without a substantial change in funding mechanisms and review processes that are sensitive to the unique aspects of Indigenous cultures we will continue to lag behind in evidence-based prevention and treatment research.
3. The continued emphasis on Indigenous research ethics and community based participatory research treating Indigenous communities as equal partners with unique cultural expertise.

4. Immediate funding for innovative recruitment and training programs for Indigenous advanced mental health professionals and researchers across all disciplines (e.g., psychiatry, psychology, sociology, and social work). Even if we began immediately, we are years away from a strong cohort of well-trained, experienced Indigenous mental health professionals and researchers.

5. Invest in and evaluate the effectiveness of innovative treatment options such as live interactive videoconferencing that provides professional psychiatric care to rural and remote Indigenous communities for children and families (Savin, Garry, Zuccaro, & Novins, 2006).

6. Increase funding for cultural programs in schools with significant Indigenous student populations to increase school adjustment and cultural identity.

As Walkup and Barlow point out, we know enough to act and to delay is to place additional generations at risk. There are costs involved, but we can pay now through effective evidence-based interventions or pay later through health services and criminal justice burden. Whatever the solutions, they will build upon cultural knowledge with strong cultural partners. As one Indigenous services provider told us

> I think there's a loss of their identity. From being Native, we lost a lot of that... parents don't teach their kids what we were taught. And once they're (kids) growing up they, they wonder, "who am I?" They're lost, you know. We need to get that back to help our people. That's what I see. They need elder's help, to teach us, then we can teach our kids. That's what's missing, that's what we need.

Acknowledgment This research was funded by the National Institute on Drug Abuse (DA13580) and the National Institute of Mental Health (MH67281), Les B. Whitbeck, Principal Investigator.

References

American Association of Medical Colleges. (2005). *Minorities in medical education: Facts and figures 2005*. Washington, DC: Author.

Angold, A., & Costello, E. (2001). Epidemiology of depression in children and adolescents. In L. Goodyer (Ed.), *The depressed child and adolescent* (2nd ed.). London: Cambridge University Press.

Bachman, R. (1992). *Death and violence on the reservation*. New York: Auburn House.

Barlow, A., & Walkup, J. (2008). The first Americans have much to teach us. *Journal of the American Academy of Child and Adolescent Psychiatry, 47*, 843–844.

Beals, J., Manson, S. M., Mitchell, C. M., & AI-SUPERPFP Team. (2003). Cultural specificity and comparison in psychiatric epidemiology: Walking the tightrope in American Indian research. *Culture, Medicine and Psychiatry, 27*, 259–289.

Beals, J., Manson, S., Whitesell, N., Spicer, P., Novins, D., Mitchell, D., et al. (2005). Prevalence of DSM-IV Disorders and attendant help-seeking in 2 American Indian reservation populations. *Archives of General Psychiatry, 62*, 99–108.

Beals, J., Piasecki, J., Nelson, S., Jones, M., Keane, E., Dauphinais, P., et al. (1997). Psychiatric disorder among American Indian adolescents: Prevalence in Northern Plains youth. *Journal of the American Academy of Child and Adolescent Psychiatry, 36*, 1252–1259.

Beauvais, F. (1980). *Preventing drug abuse among Native American young people*. Fort Collins, CO: Colorado State University.

Beauvais, F. (1998). Cultural identification and substance use in North America – An annotated bibliography. *Substance Use and Misuse, 33*(6), 1315–1336.

Billings, A., & Moos, R. (1983). Psychosocial processes of recovery among alcoholics and their families: Implications for clinicians and program evaluators. *Addictive Behaviors, 8*, 205–218.

Bureau of Indian Affairs. (2002). Federally recognized tribes. *Federal Register, 67*, 46327–46333. Retrieved November 20, 2010, from http://www.artnatam.com/tribes.html

Conger, R. (1997). The social context of substance abuse: A developmental perspective. In E. Robinson, Z. Sloboda, E. Boyd, L. Beatty, & N. Kozel (Eds.), *Rural substance abuse: State of knowledge and issues* (NIH Publication No. 97-4177, pp. 6–36). Washington, DC: NIDA.

Conger, R., Lorenz, F., Elder, G., Melby, J., Simons, R., & Conger, K. (1991). A process model of family economic pressure and early adolescent alcohol use. *Journal of Early Adolescence, 11*, 430–449.

Costa, F., Jessor, R., Donovan, J., & Fortenberry, J. (1995). Early initiation of sexual intercourse: The influence of psychosocial unconventionality. *Journal of Research on Adolescence, 5*, 93–121.

Costello, E., Farmer, E., Angold, A., Burns, B., & Erkanli, A. (1997). Psychiatric disorders among American Indian and white youth in Appalachia: The great Smokey mountain study. *American Journal of Public Health, 87*, 827–832.

Crawford, D., Cheadle, J., & Whitbeck, L. (2009). *Tribal vs. public schools: Perceived discrimination and school adjustment among Indigenous children from early to mid-adolescence. Journal of American Indian Education, in press.*

Department of Health and Human Services. (2009). *The 2008 HHS poverty guidelines: One version of the [US] Federal poverty measure.* Retrieved November 10, 2009, from http://aspe.hhs.gov/poverty/08Poverty.shtml

Dion, K., Dion, K., & Pak, A. (1992). Personality based hardiness as a buffer for discrimination-related stress in members of Toronto's Chinese community. *Canadian Journal of Behavioral Science, 24*, 517–536.

Gone, J. (2003). American Indian mental health service delivery: Persistent challenges and future prospects. In J. Mio & G. Iwamasa (Eds.), *Culturally diverse mental health: The challenges of research and resistance* (pp. 211–229). New York: Brunner-Routledge.

Gone, J. (2004). Mental health services for Native Americans in the 21st century United States. *Profession Psychology: Research and Practice, 35*, 10–18.

Government Accountability Office. (2005). *Indian health service: Health care services are not always available to Native Americans.* Report to the Committee on Indian Health Affairs, US Senate.

Gray, N., & Nye, P. (2001). American Indian and Alaska Native substance abuse: Co-morbidity and cultural issues. *American Indian/Alaska Native Mental Health Research Journal, 23*, 67–84.

Gregory, R., Abello, A., & Johnson, J. (1996). The individual economic well-being of Native American men and women during the 1980s: A decade of moving backwards. In G. Sandefur, R. Rindfuss, & B. Rohen (Eds.), *Changing numbers, changing needs: American Indian demography and public health* (pp. 133–171). Washington, DC: National Academy Press.

Herman-Stahl, M., Spencer, D., & Duncan, J. (2003). The implications of cultural orientation for substance use among American Indians. *American Indian and Alaska Native Mental Health Research, 11*, 46–66.

Hobson, C., Delunas, L., & Kesic, D. (2001). Compelling evidence of the need for corporate work/life balance initiatives: Results from a national survey of stressful life-events. *Journal of Employment Counseling, 38*, 38–44.

Hoge, D., Smit, E., & Hanson, S. (1990). School experiences predicting changes in self-esteem of sixth- and seventh-grade students. *Journal of Educational Psychology, 82*(1), 117–127.

Indian Health Service. (1992). *The state of Native American youth health.* Washington, DC: Indian Services.

Indian Health Service. (2006). *Strategic plan 2006–2011*. Retrieved March 11, 2009, from http://www.ihs.gov/NonMedicalPrograms/PlanningEvaluation/documents/IHSStrategicPlan 20062011.pdf

Indian Health Service. (2009). *IHS fact sheets: Indian health disparities*. Retrieved December 10, 2009, from http://info.ihs.gov/Disparities

Jessor, R., & Jessor, S. (1977). *Problem behavior and psychosocial development*. New York: Academic Press.

Jones, D. (2006). Public health then and now: The persistence of American Indian health disparities. *American Journal of Public Health, 96*, 2122–2134.

Kessler, R. (1994a). Building on the ECA: The National Comorbidity Survey and the children's ECA. *International Journal of Methods in Psychiatric Research, 4*, 81–94.

Kessler, R. (1994b). The National Comorbidity Survey of the United States. *International Review of Psychiatry, 6*, 365–376.

Kessler, R., Berglund, P., Demler, O., Jin, R., & Walters, E. (2005). Lifetime prevalence and age-of-onset distributions of DSM-IV disorders in the National Comorbidity Survey Replication. *Archives of General Psychiatry, 62*, 593–602.

Kessler, R., Mickelson, K., & Williams, D. (1999). The prevalence, distribution, and mental health correlates of perceived discrimination in the United States. *Journal of Health and Social Behavior, 40*, 208–230.

Krieger, N., & Sidney, S. (1996). Racial discrimination and blood pressure: The CARDIA study of young black and white women and men. *American Journal of Public Health, 86*, 1370–1378.

LaFromboise, T., Hoyt, D., Oliver, L., & Whitbeck, L. (2006). Family, community, and school influences on resilience among American Indian adolescents in the upper Midwest. *Journal of Community Psychology, 34*, 193–209.

Leland, J. (1980). Native American alcohol use: A review of the literature. In P. D. Mail & D. R. MacDonald (Eds.), *Tulapai to Takay: A bibliography of alcohol use and abuse among Native American of North America* (pp. 1–56). New Haven, CT: HRAF.

Loeber, R., Farrington, D., Stouthamer-Loeber, M., & Van Kammern, W. (1998). *Antisocial behavior and mental health problems: Explanatory factors in childhood and adolescence*. Mahwah, NJ: Erlbaum.

Lysne, M., & Levy, G. (1997). Differences in ethnic identity in Native American adolescents as a function of school context. *Journal of Adolescent Research, 12*, 372–388.

Manataka American Indian Council. (2009). Retrieved November 20, 2009, from http://www.manataka.org/page237.html

Manson, S., Beals, J., Klein, S., & Croy, C. (2005). Social epidemiology of trauma among two American Indian reservation populations. *American Journal of Public Health, 95*, 851–859.

Manson, S., Shore, J., & Bloom, J. (1985). The depressive experience in American Indian communities: A challenge for psychiatric theory and diagnosis. In A. Kleinman & B. Good (Eds.), *Culture and depression* (pp. 331–338). Berkeley, CA: University of California Press.

Moncher, M., Holden, G., & Trimble, J. (1990). Substance abuse among Native-American youth. *Journal of Consulting and Clinical Psychology, 58*, 408–415.

Noe, T., Fleming, C., & Manson, S. (2003). Healthy nations: Reducing substance abuse in American Indian & Alaska Native community. *Journal of Psychoactive Drugs, 35*, 15–25.

Ogunwole, S. (2006). *We the people: American Indians and Alaska Natives in the United States* (Census 2000 Special Reports (CENSR-28)). Washington, DC: U.S. Department of Commerce, Economics and Statistics Administration.

Ovaschel, H. (1983). Maternal depression and child dysfunction: Children at risk. In B. B. Lahey & A. E. Kazdin (Eds.), *Advances in clinical child psychology*. New York: Plenum Press.

Phinney, J. (1989). Stages of ethnic identity development in minority group adolescents. *Journal of Early Adolescence, 9*, 34–49.

Phinney, J., & Alipuria, L. (1990). Ethnic identity in older adolescents from four ethnic groups. *Journal of Adolescence, 13*, 171–183.

Roeser, R., Eccles, J., & Sameroff, A. (2000). School as a context of early adolescents' academic and social-emotional development: A summary of research findings. *The Elementary School Journal, 100*, 443–471.

Sampson, R., & Laub, J. (1993). *Crime in the making: Pathways and turning points through life*. Cambridge, MA: Harvard University Press.

Sandefur, G., Rindfuss, R., & Cohen, B. (1996). *Changing numbers, changing needs: American Indian demography and public health*. Washington, DC: National Academy Press.

Savin, D., Garry, M., Zuccaro, P., & Novins, D. (2006). Telepsychiatry for treating rural American Indian youth. *Journal of the American Academy of Child and Adolescent Psychiatry, 45*, 484–488.

Spicer, P., Beals, J., Croy, C., Mitchell, C., Novins, D., Moore, L., et al. (2003). The prevalence of DSM-III-R alcohol dependence in two American Indian populations. *Alcoholism Clinical and Experimental Research, 27*, 1785–1797.

Spicer, P., Novins, D., Mitchell, C., & Beals, J. (2003). Aboriginal social organization, contemporary experience and American Indian adolescent alcohol use. *Journal of Studies on Alcohol, 64*, 450–457.

Steinberg, L. (1996). *Beyond the classroom: Why school reform has failed and what parents need to do*. New York: Simon & Schuster.

Substance Abuse and Mental Health Services Administration. (2006). *Results from the 2005 national survey on drug use and health: National findings*. Retrieved February 20, 2009, from http://www.oas.samhsa.gov/NSDUH/2k5NSDUH/2k5Results.htm

Thompson, V. (1996). Perceived experiences of racism as stressful life events. *Community Mental Health, 32*, 223–233.

Topper, M. (1980). Drinking as an expression of status: Navajo male adolescents. In J. Waddell & M. Everett (Eds.), *Indian drinking in the southwest*. Tucson, AZ: University of Arizona Press.

Torres-Stone, R., Whitbeck, L., Chen, X., Johnson, K., & Olson, D. (2006). Traditional practices, traditional spirituality, and alcohol cessation among American Indians. *Journal of Studies on Alcohol, 67*, 236–245.

Trimble, J., Manson, S., Dinges, N., & Medicine, B. (1984). American Indian concepts of mental health: Reflections and directions. In P. Pederson, N. Sartorius, & A. Marsella (Eds.), *Mental health services: The cross-cultural context* (pp. 199–220). Beverly Hills, CA: Sage.

Trosper, R. (1996). American Indian poverty on reservations. In G. Sandefur, R. Rindfuss, & B. Cohen (Eds.), *Changing numbers, changing needs: American Indian demography and public health* (pp. 172–195). Washington, DC: National Academy Press.

US Department of Health and Human Services. (2001). *Mental health: Culture, race, and ethnicity – A supplement to mental health: A report of the surgeon general*. Rockville, MD: US Department of Health and Human Services, Substance Abuse and Mental Health Services Administration, Center for Mental Health Services.

Vega, W., Gil, A., & Zimmerman, R. (1993). Patterns of drug use among Cuban-American, African-American, and White non-Hispanic boys. *American Journal of Public Health, 83*, 257–259.

Walls, M., Johnson, K., Whitbeck, L., & Hoyt, D. (2006). Mental health and substance abuse services preferences among American Indian people of the Northern Midwest. *Community Mental Health Journal, 42*, 521–535.

Weibel, J. (1982). Native American Indians, urbanization and alcohol: A developing urban Native American drinking ethos. In NIAAA (Ed.), *Alcohol and health monograph* (No. 4, DHHS Publication No. ADM 82-1193, pp. 331–358). Washington, DC: US Department of Health and Human Services.

Westmoreland, T., & Watson, K. (2006). Fulfilling the hollow promises made to Indigenous people: Redeeming hollow promises: The case for mandatory spending on health care for American Indians and Alaska Natives. *American Journal of Public Health, 96*, 600–605.

Whitbeck, L., Chen, X., Hoyt, D., & Adams, G. (2004). Discrimination, historical loss, and enculturation: Culturally specific risk and resiliency factors for alcohol abuse among American Indians. *Journal of Alcohol Studies, 65*, 409–418.

Whitbeck, L., Hoyt, D., Chen, X., & Johnson, K. (2006). Prevalence and comorbidity of mental disorders among American Indian adults in the Northern Midwest. *Journal of Adolescent Health, 39*, 427–434.

Whitbeck, L., Hoyt, D., & Johnson, K. (2006). Prevalence and comorbidity of mental disorders among American Indian children in the Northern Midwest. *Social Psychiatry and Epidemiology, 41*, 632–640.

Whitbeck, L., Hoyt, D., Stubben, J., & LaFromboise, T. (2001). Traditional culture and academic success among American Indian children in the Upper Midwest. *Journal of American Indian Education, 40*, 48–60.

Whitbeck, L., Johnson, K., Hoyt, D., & Walls, M. (2006). Mental health and substance abuse services preferences among American Indian people of the Northern Midwest. *Journal of Adolescent Health, 39*, 427–434.

Whitbeck, L., McMorris, B., Hoyt, D., Stubben, J., & LaFromboise, T. (2002). Perceived discrimination, traditional practices, and depressive symptoms among American Indians in the Upper Midwest. *Journal of Health and Social Behavior, 43*, 400–418.

Whitbeck, L., Yu, M., Johnson, K., Hoyt, D., & Walls, M. (2008). Diagnostic prevalence rates from early to mid-adolescence among indigenous adolescents: First results from a longitudinal study. *Journal of American Academy of Child and Adolescent Psychiatry, 47*, 890–900.

Williams, D., Spencer, M., & Jackson, J. (1999). Race, stress, and physical health. In J. Contrada & R. Ashmore (Eds.), *Self, social identity, and physical health* (pp. 71–100). New York: Oxford University Press.

Williams, D., & Williams-Morris, R. (2000). Racism and mental health: The African American experience. *Ethnicity & Health, 5*, 243–268.

Williams, D., Yu, Y., & Jackson, J. S. (1997). Racial differences in physical and mental health. *Journal of Health Psychology, 2*, 335–351.

Yoder, K., Whitbeck, L., Hoyt, D., & LaFromboise, T. (2006). Suicide ideation among American Indian youths. *Archives of Suicide Research, 10*, 177–190.

Zimmerman, M., Ramirez, J., Washienko, K., Walter, B., & Dyer, S. (1998). Enculturation hypothesis: Exploring direct and protective effects among Native American youth. In H. I. McCubbin, E. A. Thompson, A. I. Thompson, & J. E. Fromer (Eds.), *Resiliency in Native American and immigrant families* (pp. 199–220). Thousand Oaks, CA: Sage.

Understanding the Hispanic Health Paradox Through a Multi-Generation Lens: A Focus on Behavior Disorders

William A. Vega and William M. Sribney

Overview

The Hispanic Health Paradox refers to the usual finding in population health studies that the most vulnerable sub-population of immigrants actually have superior morbidity and mortality compared to either the US population or Hispanics born in the United States. In this paper we examine this paradox using an epidemiologic strategy of scrutinizing inter-generational change processes in the Latino population.

The Hispanic Health Paradox is especially marked for morbidity and mortality in people of Mexican origin who number about 28 million of 47 million total Latinos residing in United States during 2009. Given that nearly half of the US Mexican origin population is of foreign birth, the health status differences of the foreign- and US-born nativity groups is of profound interest. Attention in recent reviews has been given to the quality of the data relied upon to study differences in morbidity and mortality rates, the extent to which this is an enduring phenomena or a secular trend, and to discovering determinants that act as risk and protective factors for respective disease outcomes leading to health disparities (Arias, Eschbach, Schauman, Backlund, & Sorlie, 2009; Palloni & Arias, 2004; Vega, Rodriguez, & Gruskin, 2009).

Marked differences in estimated rates of behavioral health problems are especially noticeable in comparing nativity differences of Mexican origin people (Vega et al., 1998) Common mental health and substance abuse problems pose an important population burden of disease, and rates for these medically significant problems are markedly lower among immigrants when compared to US born of Mexican origin in population studies (Alegria et al., 2007, 2008). It may be that these behavioral lifestyle problems are among the most susceptible to change under conditions of rapid resocialization of families who confront adaptive stresses associated with immigration in their children. Ninety-five percent of children of immigrants

W.A. Vega (✉)
Edward R. Roybal Institute on Aging, University of Southern California (USC), USC Roybal Institute, Montgomery Ross Fisher Building, Los Angeles, CA 90089-0411, USA
e-mail: williaav@usc.edu

G. Carlo et al. (eds.), *Health Disparities in Youth and Families*, Nebraska Symposium on Motivation 57, DOI 10.1007/978-1-4419-7092-3_7, © Springer Science+Business Media, LLC 2011

are US born, which suggests that selective environmental exposures that differ between parents and children may play a formative role in the pathogenesis of these addictive and non-addictive mental health and behavioral problems (Vega & Gil, 1998). Almost 100 years ago similar observations were made by sociologists of the Chicago School that were observing the transitions in problem behaviors occurring inter-generationally among immigrant families from Mexico, as well as Southern and Eastern Europe who were settling in the slums of the central city (Sutherland, 1934).

More recent research has reported that addictive and non-addictive disorders are inter-related, that is to say they frequently co-occur in the same person (Vega, Canino, Cao, & Alegria, 2009). A common pattern is for non-addictive mental health problems to appear first followed by addictive behaviors, but there is considerable variation. Nonetheless, it is clear from current evidence that immigrants are less vulnerable to these types of behavior problems and if they do experience them they tend to do so if they arrived in the United States during childhood, with a far lower probability of exhibiting these behaviors if they arrived during early adulthood or thereafter. The major shift in risk is noticeable in the second and third generations post immigration. Thus, the Hispanic Health Paradox has provoked the search for explanations regarding why and how this unfolding of risk and pathologic outcomes occurs, and more importantly how can it be restrained? The search for determinants and modifiable protective factors has been hampered by the complexity of an issue that involves social, cultural, biological, and economic determinants, and which must be reconciled theoretically and empirically (Zambrana & Carter-Pokras, 2009).

Developing sound explanations and testing hypotheses requires good quality data sets. The necessary data qualities include sufficiently wide topic coverage among data elements and adequate technical characteristics including sample and subsample size adequacy to permit close scrutiny of underlying processes involved in the generative processes of behavioral disorders on a population level. There are many limitations that have made this difficult in past years, including inadequate sampling of the Hispanic population to permit the understanding of differences in population risk by markers such as language, nativity, national origin, region, sex, age, etc., as well as theoretically relevant life history information, comprehensive health and mental health inventories, and information about lifestyle factors. In addition, the absence of large studies, until very recently, that included Spanish language samples, and time ordered data, were also formidable obstacles, and some continue to persist. Over time many of these problems have been partially or wholly overcome in recent decades as public heath experts have realized the importance of the Hispanic population in terms of their demographic impact on the nation and the lessons to be learned about how health disparities emerge and potentially remedied from careful scientific investigations.

Despite limitations inherent to our information sources, a body of relatively recent large scale research has been completed that permits a more advanced level of analysis for deriving insights into putatively causal processes. The accumulation of evidence, including findings from large population studies in Mexico and

Latin America, has provided an opportunity to evaluate and refine observations from earlier research, and to begin to distinguish the unique paths of social adaptation and social adjustment that have resulted in distinct Hispanic nationality and social-demographic groups having different level of risks for behavioral problems as their social histories play out in the United States.

Understanding Underlying Patterns of Accelerated Risk

It has been evident since the mid-1980s and with the publication of the Hispanic Health and Nutrition Examination Survey (HHANES) results in a special Supplement of the American Journal of Public Health (Vol. 80) in 1990, that immigrants had lower rates of key cause-specific mortality indicators such as cancer and heart disease. The HHANES reported rates for two important behavioral health problems, major depression and substance abuse, and in both instances the same pattern held as reported for disease-specific causes of mortality: foreign birth was associated with significantly lower rates (Amaro, Whitaker, Coffman, & Heeren, 1990; Moscicki, Locke, Rae, & Boyd, 1989). In the ensuing years several national studies confirmed these early impressions with far more detail and a wider range of behavioral problems. One of the most important findings that helped explain differences in population rates was that immigrants generally had the first manifestations (onsets) of serious behavioral health problems at a later age than US-born Latinos and these usually occurred after immigration, a pattern that results in lower rates of population prevalence between nativity groups (Vega & Sribney, 2009).

Other comprehensive population surveys with adequate coverage of Latinos and behavior health problems that were medically relevant, including data on Mexican Americans used for the presentation in this review, include (in chronologic order), the Los Angeles Epidemiologic Catchment Area Project in the 1980s, the Mexican American Prevalence and Services Survey in the 1990s, and two surveys, the National Epidemiologic Survey on Alcohol and Related Conditions, and the National Latino and Asian American Survey, completed during the current decade from 2000–2009 (Alegria et al., 2007, 2008; Grant et al., 2004; Karno, Hough, Burnam, Escobar, & Telles, 1987; Vega et al., 1998). A compilation of results from these studies can be found elsewhere, however, these studies consistently found medically significant substance use disorders to be higher in US-born Latinos, especially for Mexican Americans. Examination of data for smaller Latino ethnic subgroups for which survey data are now available shows the largest deviation from the paradox occurs among Puerto Ricans. This is likely because they are not immigrants in the formal sense as birth in Puerto Rico carries with it US citizenship, and English language and American culture are part of the socialization process on the island. Puerto Ricans born on the island arrive in the US at an earlier age than other subgroups and become English dominant speakers more quickly than do other Latino subgroups. This reflects both experiencing significant pre-socialization in Puerto Rico and early life resettlement, and these factors seemingly contribute to a unique pattern of generally higher risk for many health related conditions in the United States. Puerto Ricans born in Puerto Rico, nonetheless, have lower rates compared to the White non-Hispanic population of the US.

The results of these studies are remarkable and also enigmatic. Historical studies of mental health and international immigration to the US and Europe reveal research with dramatically different conclusions, and their findings report much higher rates of psychiatric hospitalizations for immigrants than for other native born residents. The issue became so notable 80 years ago that it resulted in a wave of national legislation to imposed stricter limits on immigration quotas to the US (Portes & Rumbaut, 1990). Even today, UK and European researchers continue to report higher rates of psychiatric disorders among immigrants, whether they are migrating among European nations or originating from other continents (Vega & Lewis-Fernandez, 2008). Thus the scientific mystery persists and the search for substantive and methodological explanations will also continue until reasonable integration of findings and explanations is attained.

Migration and Genetic Adaptation to New Environments

Richard Cooper presented a seminal explanation that he called the "context-dependence" model designed to illustrate how latent genetic liability emerges for complex diseases specifically when people are transplanted from one social and physical environment to another as occurs consequent to international migration (Cooper, 2003). His model was designed to provide a heuristic for understanding differences in rates of hypertensive disorder (or similar complex diseases involving multiple genes) in West Africa in comparison to African Americans in the US who likely had their continental origins in the latter region. The key mechanism described in the model is that latent dispositions of specific gene mutations that create a liability for a disease, that remained unexpressed in the region of population origin, may be expressed in a new environment through gene–environment (G × E) interplay. This process potentially results in abnormal functional changes in genes leading to pathogenic pathways for individuals who carry these specific gene mutations—leading to a phenotype (hypertension) in this analog.

The Cooper model is instructive for thinking about the emergence of risk for substance related problems among people of Mexican origin in the US. National population rates of addictive disorders in Mexico are very low and comparable to the rates reported in the US among recently arrived immigrants from Mexico in their first decade or so of US residence (Medina-Mora et al., 2005; Vega, Alderete, Kolody, & Aguilar-Gaxiola, 1998). In the US general population, the process of addiction at the individual level is also selective, and only 1 in 10 people who use addictive drugs are believed to become dependent and habitual users. While it is certainly probable that people develop lifestyles that produce vulnerabilities to disease as a sole consequence of changes in behavioral socialization in a new social environment (such as overeating and alcohol and tobacco use), it is also probable that risk for behavioral health problems is disproportionate for individuals that have genetically derived traits that are heritable such as temperament. Logically, risk for behavioral problems is likely greater for individuals with maladaptive responses to life stress and trauma as well. As recommended by the Institute of Medicine, these possible linkages are now widely pursued and investigated in behavioral research and add an important new dimension to social epidemiologic explanations of complex diseases (Hernandez & Blazer, 2006).

Objectives of the Review

As noted, few large field studies have been designed to address key questions of interest regarding patterns and determinants of Latino population differences in health and behavioral health. My colleagues and I had an opportunity to conduct such an investigation and were able to draw representative samples that were of sufficient size to permit detailed analyses, albeit not as comprehensive as we would consider optimal. Below we present work that provides important insights on intergenerational patterns in behavioral health among Mexican origin people that have not been previously presented in any other published research of which we are aware, and that we believe can stimulate further advances in future research studies of the paradox.

Methods

A detailed methodological description of the methods and design of the Mexican American Prevalence and Services Survey (MAPSS) can be found in Vega, Kolody, et al. (1998). The MAPSS sample is a representative sample of 3,012 Mexican-origin adults aged 18–59 years from the Fresno, California, Metropolitan Statistical Area (MSA). The sample was selected under a fully probabilistic stratified, multi-stage cluster design. Face-to-face field interviewing was conducted in 1995–1996, and the response rate was 90% among screened eligible households.

The diagnostic protocol used in the MAPSS was the Composite International Diagnostic Interview (CIDI) (Kessler et al., 1994), a fully structured clinical inventory using DSM-III-R diagnostic criteria, which was administered by trained lay interviewers. Information about parents' mental health and substance abuse problems were asked within the nondiagnostic sections of the interview. There were four core questions asked about biological fathers and mothers separately, these were: (1) *Did your biological father/mother ever have periods lasting 2 weeks or more when he/she was depressed or down in the dumps most of the time?* (2) *Did your biological father/mother have periods of a month or more when he/she was constantly nervous, edgy, or anxious?* (3) *Did your biological father/mother have a problem with drinking?* and (4) *Did he/she ever have a problem with illegal drugs?* The first question in this series had as a possible response, *No knowledge about father/mother*, and if this response was given, the subsequent questions were not asked.

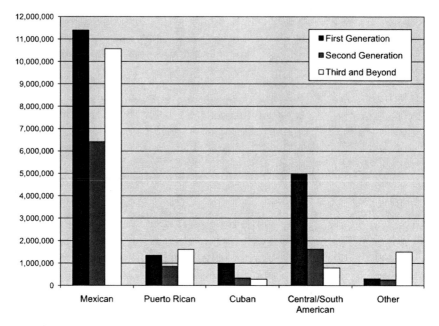

Fig. 1 US Latino population by national origin: Average for years 2004–2008. (Source: Merged Current Population Survey (CPS) annual demographic files, 2004–2008.)

Figure 1 was produced using data from the Current Population Survey (US Census, 2008). Totals in the figure are US national averages for the years 2004–2008. All percentages reported in Table 1 and Figs. 2–13 are weighted proportions from the MAPSS survey. All inferential procedures used accounted for the complex survey design. Analyses were conducted using Stata statistical software version 10.1 (Stata, 2008).

Results

Figure 1 gives recent population totals of Latinos in the US by national origin. Two-thirds (66%) of all the Latinos in the US are Mexican origin, followed by Latinos of Central and South American origin (17%). Latinos of Puerto Rican (9%) and Cuban (4%) origin are a relatively small proportion of the total. Proportions by national origin for immigrants (first generation) are similar: Mexicans (60%) and Central and South Americans (26%) together comprise the vast majority of all Latino immigrants in the US. Puerto Ricans (7%) and Cubans (5%) again only form a small proportion of the total. (Puerto Ricans are, of course, US citizens, and for them, the terms "immigrant" and "US born" in this article refer to island versus mainland birthplace.)

Table 1 Sample ($N = 3,012$) characteristics[a] of Mexican-origin adults (ages 18–59) from the MAPSS (Fresno County, California) survey, with prevalence of DSM-III-R alcohol abuse or dependence and drug abuse or dependence

	Immigrants			US born		
	Female	Male	Total	Female	Male	Total
Sample size (N)	912	922	1,834	604	574	1,178
Weighted percentage	44.8	55.2	60.1	49.4	50.6	39.9
Education (years):						
0–6	55.3	47.1	50.8	2.1	5.1	3.6
7–11	28.1	32.6	30.6	43.9	35.2	39.5
12	10.2	9.8	10.0	29.7	31.3	30.5
≥13	6.4	10.4	8.6	24.2	28.4	26.3
Family income ($):						
<6,000	15.8	13.3	14.4	7.0	7.3	7.2
6,000–11,999	42.3	32.1	36.7	25.8	19.6	22.6
12,000–17,999	27.1	28.3	27.8	24.6	22.8	23.7
18,000–35,999	10.4	17.2	14.2	25.1	24.2	24.7
≥36,000	4.3	9.1	7.0	17.6	26.0	21.9
Language preference:						
Spanish all of the time	59.7	46.3	52.3	2.9	5.2	4.1
Spanish most of the time	15.6	18.0	16.9	6.3	5.0	5.7
Spanish and English equally	21.1	28.1	24.9	24.1	22.8	23.4
English most of the time	3.2	6.2	4.9	33.8	44.9	39.4
English all of the time	0.4	1.5	1.0	32.9	22.1	27.5
Alcohol abuse or dependence, lifetime	1.5	15.8	9.4	13.7	30.4	22.1
Drug abuse or dependence, lifetime	1.4	4.7	3.2	8.8	18.4	13.7

[a] All data except sample counts are reported as weighted percentages.

Table 1 shows the sample characteristics of the MAPSS survey, a representative sample of Mexican-origin adults (ages 18–59) residing in central California (Fresno County). Immigrants made up about 60% of the sample, and among immigrants the majority (55%) were men, whereas among the US born, men and women were represented in roughly equal proportions. Immigrants had appreciably lower levels of education than the US born, with 51% of immigrants having 6 years or less of education compared to 4% of the US born. Differences in income between immigrants and the US born were not as extreme as differences in education, but they were still largely different with immigrants having much lower incomes. As one would expect, far greater numbers (52%) of immigrants preferred to speak Spanish all of the time compared to the US born (4%). However, only 28% of the US born preferred English all of the time, and about equal proportions of immigrants (25%) and the US born (23%) stated that between Spanish and English, they did not prefer one language over the other.

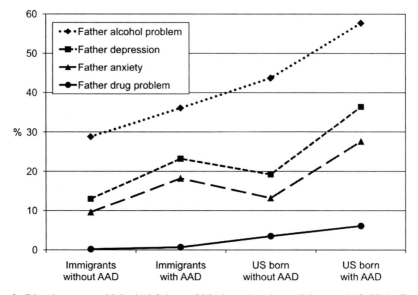

Fig. 2 Disorders among biological fathers of Mexican-American adults (aged 18–59) in Fresno County, California, with or without alcohol abuse or dependence (AAD) by nativity

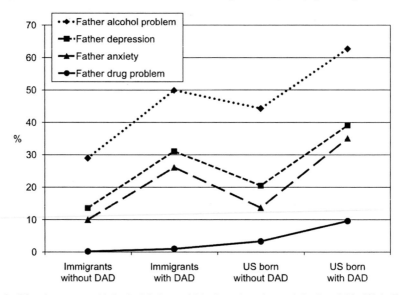

Fig. 3 Disorders among biological fathers of Mexican-American adults (aged 18–59) in Fresno County, California, with or without drug abuse or dependence (DAD) by nativity

Table 1 also gives the lifetime prevalence of alcohol and drug abuse or dependence among Mexican-origin adults in this survey. Prevalences of alcohol and drug disorders were extremely low among immigrant women (less than 2%). Immigrant men and US-born women had similar levels of alcohol abuse or dependence (16 and

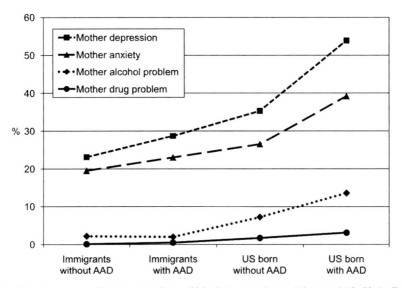

Fig. 4 Disorders among biological mothers of Mexican-American adults (aged 18–59) in Fresno County, California, with or without alcohol abuse or dependence (AAD) by nativity

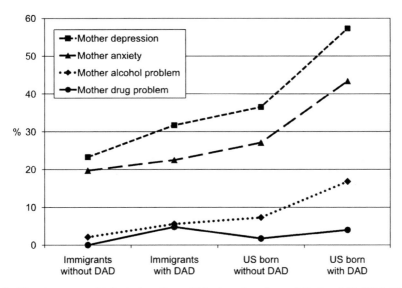

Fig. 5 Disorders among biological mothers of Mexican-American adults (aged 18–59) in Fresno County, California, with or without drug abuse or dependence (DAD) by nativity

14%, respectively); however, US-born women had higher levels of drug abuse or dependence (9%) compared to immigrant men (5%). US-born men had by far the greatest levels of both alcohol and drug disorders: 30% had an alcohol disorder at some point in their life and 9% had a drug disorder.

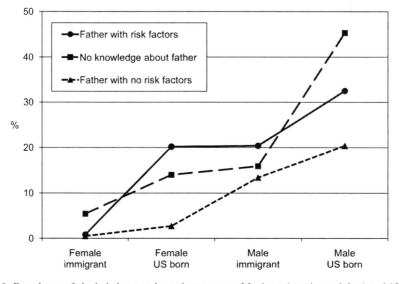

Fig. 6 Prevalence of alcohol abuse or dependence among Mexican-American adults (aged 18–59) in Fresno County, California, by risk factors of fathers

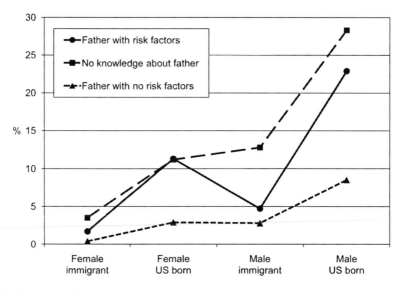

Fig. 7 Prevalence of drug abuse or dependence among Mexican-American adults (aged 18–59) in Fresno County, California, by risk factors of fathers

Figures 2 and 3 give the prevalence of mental health and substance-use problems in fathers of MAPSS survey respondents, as reported by the respondent. Figure 2 divides respondents by lifetime alcohol abuse or dependence (AAD) status and by nativity. Figure 3 categorizes respondents by drug abuse or dependence (DAD) diagnosis as well as nativity. Among US-born Mexican-Americans with alcohol abuse or

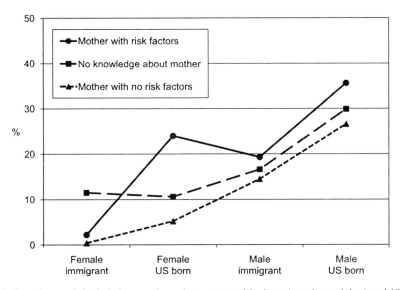

Fig. 8 Prevalence of alcohol abuse or dependence among Mexican-American adults (aged 18–59) in Fresno County, California, by risk factors of mothers

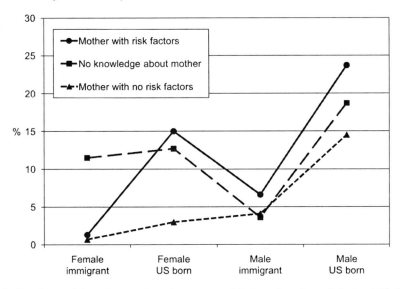

Fig. 9 Prevalence of drug abuse or dependence among Mexican-American adults (aged 18–59) in Fresno County, California, by risk factors of mothers

dependence, 60% reported that their biological father had an alcohol problem, 36% reported that their father had periods of depression, 28% reported that their father had problems with anxiety, and 6% reported their father had a problem with illegal drugs. All of the levels of these problems in fathers, except for drugs, were significantly higher among the US born with alcohol abuse or dependence compared to

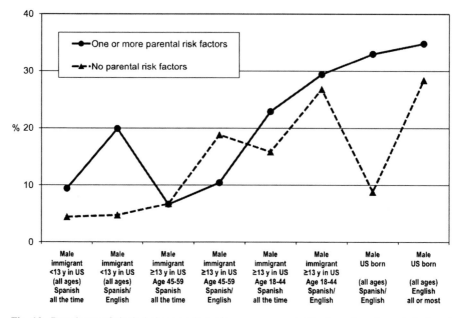

Fig. 10 Prevalence of alcohol abuse or dependence among male Mexican-American adults (aged 18–59) in Fresno County, California, by risk factors of parents, age, nativity, time in US for immigrants, and language

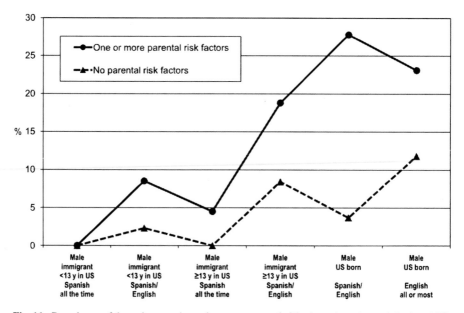

Fig. 11 Prevalence of drug abuse or dependence among male Mexican-American adults (aged 18–44) in Fresno County, California, by risk factors of parents, nativity, time in US for immigrants, and language

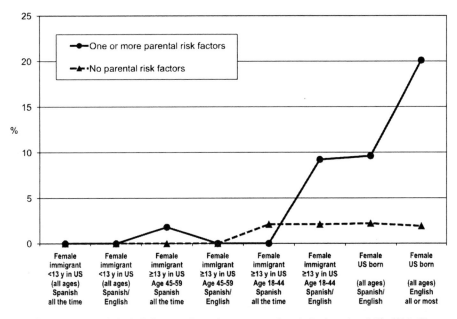

Fig. 12 Prevalence of alcohol abuse or dependence among female Latinas (aged 18–59) in Fresno County, California, by risk factors of parents, age, nativity, time in US for immigrants, and language

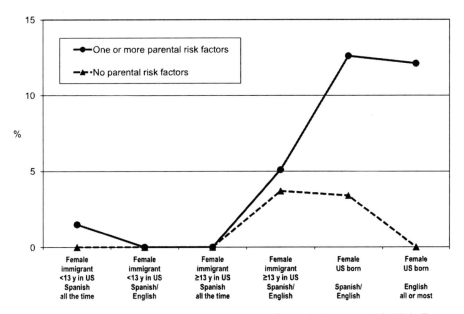

Fig. 13 Prevalence of drug abuse or dependence among female Latinas (aged 18–44) in Fresno County, California, by risk factors of parents, nativity, time in US for immigrants, and language

those without this diagnosis. Immigrants *with* AAD reported *lower* levels of alcohol and drug problems among fathers compared to the US born *without* AAD, but levels of reported depression and anxiety in fathers were similar in these two groups. Immigrants without AAD had the lowest levels of problems among their fathers.

With respondents categorized by lifetime drug abuse or dependence status, Fig. 3 reveals a very similar pattern to that in Fig. 2, with important exceptions, however. Here immigrants with DAD reported levels of depression and anxiety that were roughly 10% higher than that reported among fathers of US born without DAD, but still roughly 10% lower than that among fathers of US born with DAD.

Figures 4 and 5 are similar to Figs. 2 and 3, except that they show levels of problems among mothers. Results for mothers were similar to that among fathers. The US born with AAD or DAD report the highest levels of problems among mothers, followed by US born without AAD or DAD and immigrants with AAD or DAD, with immigrants without AAD or DAD reporting the lowest levels. The main difference in these results are that depression and anxiety were the most frequently reported problems among mothers, with alcohol and drug problems reported much less frequently than among fathers. It is notable that 57% of the US born with DAD and 54% of the US born with AAD reported depression among their mothers, which are significantly higher levels of these problems than those reported by the other respondents.

Figures 7 and 8 reverse the projections in Figs. 2 and 3. In Figs. 7 and 8, the prevalence of lifetime alcohol abuse or dependence is plotted for persons who reported one or more problems (alcohol, drug, depression, or anxiety) among their fathers, for persons who had fathers with no problems, and for persons who had no knowledge of their biological fathers. For US-born men, those with fathers with problems had much higher rates of AAD compared to those with fathers with no problems (45% versus 20%) and much higher rates of DAD (23% versus 8%). These dramatic differences, however, were not seen among immigrant men; there were no significant differences in levels of AAD or DAD between those who reported having fathers with problems compared to those with fathers with no problems.

The pattern for women was similar to that among men; US-born women who reported having fathers with problems had much higher rates of AAD compared to those with fathers with no problems (20% versus 3%) and much higher rates of DAD (11% versus 3%). Immigrant women had low levels of AAD and DAD regardless of their father's status.

Figures 8 and 9 are similar to Figs. 6 and 7, except that rates by mother's status are plotted. Results, however, are very different from those by father's status. Here, mother's status had no significant association with levels of AAD and DAD among men, whether US or foreign born. But this was not the case among US-born women. Among US-born women, mother's status was significant, with those reporting problems among mothers having higher AAD prevalence (24%) compared to those with mothers with no problems (5%) and higher DAD prevalence (15% versus 3%). Immigrant women showed no differences in AAD or DAD prevalence by mother's status. Interestingly, immigrant women who reported no knowledge of their mother had higher levels of AAD (12%) and DAD (12%) than other immigrant women (levels of 2% or less); however, because of the small numbers involved, these differences did not reach statistical significance.

Figures 10, 11, 12, and 13 expand on the results in Figs. 6, 7, 8, and 9 by plotting prevalence of AAD and DAD, not only by sex and nativity, but also by time in the US for immigrants and language preference. Problems for father or mother are combined in these figures, and rates are shown for those with one or more problems in either parent (or no knowledge of either parent) compared to those with no problems in either parent (with knowledge of both parents). For alcohol abuse or dependence, shown for men in Fig. 10 and for women in Fig. 12, long-time (≥ 13 years in US) immigrants were also divided by age (18–44 or 45–49). In Figs. 10, 11, 12, and 13, the "Spanish/English" language category is always the complement of the alternative category, which is Spanish all of the time for immigrants and English all or most of the time for the US born.

Figure 10 shows a very clear result: among Mexican-American men, parent risk factors are only associated with differences in levels of lifetime alcohol abuse or dependence for two subgroups of men. These subgroups are US-born men who preferred Spanish all or most of the time or Spanish and English equally (33% for those with parental risk factors versus 9% for those with none) and immigrant men who have resided in the US less than 13 years and who preferred a mix of Spanish and English (20% versus 5%).

Figure 11 for drug abuse or dependence among men is not as clear cut. For all subgroups (except male immigrants less than 13 years in the US who preferred Spanish all of the time), those with parental risk factors have higher levels of DAD compared to those with no parental risk factors. Consistent with Fig. 10, the biggest difference in DAD levels was seen among US-born men who preferred Spanish all or most of the time or Spanish and English equally (28% for those with parental risk factors versus 4% for those with none).

For women in Fig. 12, the results are striking: lifetime alcohol abuse or dependence rates were only appreciable among US-born women and immigrant women aged 18–44 who had resided in the US for 13 or more years and who preferred a mix of Spanish and English or English exclusively *and* who had parental risk factors. Among those women with no parental risk factors, regardless of nativity, time in the US, age, or language preference, the rate of AAD was very low: 2% or less.

Results for drug abuse or dependence among women shown in Fig. 13 are roughly consistent with results for alcohol abuse or dependence but not as dramatic. Here, US-born women with parental risk factors had significantly higher rates of DAD compared to those with no parental risk factors. For immigrants, parental risk factors revealed no association with DAD.

Conclusion

The data we have presented illustrate how risk of behavioral problems, in the social and epidemiologic sense, advance progressively across generations of Mexican-origin people residing in the United States. These processes have implications for researchers interested in various aspects of human adaptation in new environments, especially in the context of cultural change and social inequality. It also illustrates how the question of risk is clustered in family units due to unique pathways based on parent behavioral problems and their unique effects on sex-based socialization patterns. Ultimately, it is adaptive changes in family units resulting from interactions with their social environments, and in turn, family members interacting with each other that are the centerpiece of understanding population risk for behavioral problems in a life course perspective (Gil, Vega, & Biafora, 1997). Genetic liability is involved at multiple levels of family aggregation of behavioral problems, and is likely a causal factor in person-level risk for drug dependence.

It has long been noted in the psychological treatment and prevention literature pertaining to Latinos that the processes and content of socialization for parents as contrasted with their children in immigrant families differs greatly producing potential tensions and conflicts. Families without the requisite resources and dynamics to cope and provide effective parenting are vulnerable to losing control of children in their efforts to manage unacceptable behavior. Nonetheless, as our results indicate, vulnerability is an intergenerational process which begins with immigrant parents and influences the propensity for risk in their children, and progressively takes a much more serious turn toward risk for US-born parents and their children as a more complete acculturation of both generations occurs.

Today 75% of all Latinos in the US are either immigrants or their first and second generation children. With the advent of greater constraints on immigration from Mexico and Latin America, the percentage of US-born Latinos will again increase accompanied by a higher prevalence of behavioral health problems in the Latino population. We view the results from this study as building blocks for theory and for development of more finely tuned intervention modalities. It should be remembered that behavioral health problems are merely illustrative of a much larger process affecting the health of the Latino population. People with behavioral health problems are much more likely to have additional problems of poor academic performance, suboptimal social adjustment and economic stability, more health problems and use of health care resources, and ultimately higher mortally rates and earlier death. It is estimated that the Latino population will expand to 30% of the total US population by 2050. It is worth investing in research across multiple disciplines to identify modifiable determinants, conduct large scale experiments, and innovate with policy-based environmental interventions that show promise of reducing the anticipated burden of disease in the Latino population.

References

Alegria, M., Canino, G., Shrout, P. E., Woo, M., Duan, N., Vila, D., et al. (2008). Prevalence of mental illness in immigrant and non-immigrant U.S. Latino groups. *American Journal of Psychiatry, 165*, 359–369.

Alegría, M., Mulvaney-Day, N., Torres, M., Polo, A., Cao, Z., & Canino, G. (2007). Prevalence of psychiatric disorders across Latino subgroups in the United States. *American Journal of Public Health, 97*, 68–75.

Amaro, H., Whitaker, R., Coffman, G., & Heeren, T. (1990). Acculturation and marijuana and cocaine use: Findings from the HHANES 1982–84. *American Journal of Public Health*, *80*(Suppl), 54–60.

Arias, A., Eschbach, K., Schauman, W. S., Backlund, E. L., & Sorlie, P. D. (2009). The Hispanic mortality advantage and ethnic misclassification on US death certificates. *American Journal of Public Health*, *99*, doi:10.2105/AJPH.2008.135863.

Cooper, R. (2003). Gene-environment interactions and the etiology of common complex disease. *Annals of Internal Medicine*, *139*, 437–440.

Gil, A. G., Vega, W. A., & Biafora, F. (1997). Temporal influences of family structure and family risk factors on drug use initiation in a multiethnic sample of adolescent boys. *Journal of Youth and Adolescence*, *23*, 373–393.

Grant, B. F., Stinson, F. S., Hasin, D. S., Dawson, D. A., Chou, S. P., & Anderson, K. (2004). Immigration and lifetime prevalence of DSM-IV psychiatric disorders among Mexican Americans and non-Hispanic Whites in the United States. *Archives of General Psychiatry*, *61*, 1226–1233.

Hernandez, L. M., & Blazer, D. G. (2006). *Genes, behavior, and the social environment: Moving beyond the nature/nurture debate. Committee on assessing interactions, among social, behavioral, and genetic factors in health. Institute of Medicine (U.S.)*. Washington, DC: The National Academies Press.

Karno, M., Hough, R. L., Burnam, A., Escobar, J. I., & Telles, C. (1987). Lifetime prevalence of specific psychiatric disorders among Mexican Americans and non-Hispanic whites in Los Angeles. *Archives of General Psychiatry*, *44*, 695–701.

Kessler, R. C., McGongale, K. A., Zhao, S., Nerson, C. B., Hughes, M., Eshleman, S., et al. (1994). Lifetime and 12-month prevalence of DSM-III psychiatric disorders in the United States. *Archives of General Psychiatry*, *51*, 8–19.

Medina-Mora, M. E., Borges, G., Lara, C., Benjet, C., Blanco, J., Fleiz, C., et al. (2005). Prevalence, service use, and demographic correlates of 12-month DSM-IV psychiatric disorders in Mexico: Results from the Mexican National comorbidity survey. *Psychological Medicine*, *35*, 1773–1783.

Moscicki, E. K., Locke, B. Z., Rae, D. S., & Boyd, J. H. (1989). *Depressive symptoms among Mexican Americans: The Hispanic health and nutrition examination survey. American Journal of Epidemiology*, *130*, 348–360.

Palloni, A., & Arias, E. (2004). Paradox lost: Explaining the Hispanic adult mortality advantage. *Demography*, *41*, 385–415.

Portes, A., & Rumbaut, R. (1990). *Immigrant America: A portrait*. Berkeley, CA: University of California Press.

Stata (2008). *Stata Statistical Software. Version 10.1* [computer program]. College Station, TX.

Sutherland, E. H. (1934). *Principles of criminology*. Chicago: Lippincott.

US Census (2008). Current population survey. Annual Social and Economic (ASEC) March Supplement. Data files 2004–2008. Washington, DC: U.S. Census Bureau. http://www.bls.census.gov/cps_ftp.html#psmarch (Accessed 19 Nov 2009).

Vega, W. A., Alderete, E., Kolody, B., & Aguilar-Gaxiola, S. (1998). Illicit drug use among Mexican Americans in California: Effects of gender and acculturation. *Addiction*, *93*, 1839–1850.

Vega, W. A., Canino, G., Cao, Z., & Alegria, M. (2009). Prevalence and correlates of dual diagnoses in U.S. Latinos. *Drug and Alcohol Dependence*, *100*, 32–38.

Vega, W. A., & Gil, A. G. (1998). *Drug use and ethnicity in early adolescence* (pp. 125–148). New York: Plenum Press.

Vega, W. A., Kolody, B., Aguilar-Gaxiola, S., Alderete, W., Catalano, R., & Caraveo-Anduaga, J. (1998). Lifetime prevalence of DSM-III-R psychiatric disorders among urban and rural Mexican Americans in California. *Archives of General Psychiatry*, *55*, 771–778.

Vega, W. A., & Lewis-Fernandez, R. (2008). Ethnicity and variability of psychotic symptoms. *Current Psychiatry Reports*, *10*, 223–228.

Vega, W. A., Rodriguez, M., & Gruskin, E. (2009). Health disparities in the Latino population. *Epidemiologic Reviews, 31*, 99–112.

Vega, W. A., & Sribney, W. (2009). Latino population demographics, risk factors and depression: A case study of the Mexican American prevalence and services survey. In S. Aguilar-Gaxiola, T. P. Gullotta (Eds.), *Depression in Latinos: Assessment, treatment, and prevention.* New York: Springer.

Zambrana, R. E., & Carter-Pokras, O. (2009). Role of acculturation research in advancing science and practice in reducing health care disparities among Latinos. *American Journal of Public Health,* e1–e6. doi:10.2105/AJPH.2008.138826.

Index

Note: Locators followed by 'f' refer to figures referred to in that page.

G. Carlo et al. (eds.), *Health Disparities in Youth and Families*, Nebraska Symposium on Motivation 57, DOI 10.1007/978-1-4419-7092-3,
© Springer Science+Business Media, LLC 2011